The Confederate Navy
Medical Corps

The Confederate Navy Medical Corps
Organization, Personnel and Actions

GUY R. HASEGAWA

Foreword by Gary McQuarrie

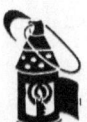

McFarland & Company, Inc., Publishers
Jefferson, North Carolina

Library of Congress Cataloguing-in-Publication Data

Names: Hasegawa, Guy R., author.
Title: The Confederate Navy Medical Corps : organization, personnel and actions / Guy R. Hasegawa.
Description: Jefferson, North Carolina : McFarland & Company, Inc., Publishers, 2024 | Includes bibliographical references and index.
Identifiers: LCCN 2024009634 | ISBN 9781476694511 (paperback : acid free paper) ♾
   ISBN 9781476652122 (ebook)
Subjects: LCSH: Confederate States of America. Navy. Medical Corps. | United States—History—Civil War, 1861-1865—Medical care. | Confederate States of America. Navy—Medical personnel. | Confederate States of America. Navy. Office of Medicine and Surgery | Confederate States of America. Navy—Registers. | Physicians—Confederate States of America—Registers. | Military planning—Medical care—Confederate States of America. | BISAC: HISTORY / Military / Naval | MEDICAL / History
Classification: LCC E625 .H387 2024 | DDC 973.7/76—dc23/eng/20230615
LC record available at https://lccn.loc.gov/2024009634

British Library cataloguing data are available

ISBN (print) 978-1-4766-9451-1
ISBN (ebook) 978-1-4766-5212-2

© 2024 Guy R. Hasegawa. All rights reserved

No part of this book may be reproduced or transmitted in any form or by any means, electronic or mechanical, including photocopying or recording, or by any information storage and retrieval system, without permission in writing from the publisher.

Front cover images: *top inset* Engraving from Joseph Becker's sketch of the hospital bombproof at Fort Fisher, North Carolina, shortly after the fort's capture by Union forces in January 1865 (*Frank Leslie's Illustrated Newspaper*, Feb. 18, 1865). CSS *Gaines* of the Confederate Navy's Mobile Squadron fought in the Battle of Mobile Bay (August 1864) and carried Passed Assistant Surgeon Osborn S. Iglehart, who kept one of the few surviving journals of medical practice aboard a Confederate vessel. Illustration by George S. Waterman, one of the vessel's midshipmen (Naval History and Heritage Command, Washington, DC, image NH 53878).

Printed in the United States of America

McFarland & Company, Inc., Publishers
   Box 611, Jefferson, North Carolina 28640
      www.mcfarlandpub.com

Contents

Foreword by Gary McQuarrie   1
Preface   5
Introduction   9

1. Beginnings of the Medical Corps   13
2. Building a Nucleus   24
3. Wanted: More Medical Officers   33
4. Standing of Naval Medical Officers   49
5. Surgeons' Stewards and Hospital Stewards   62
6. Civilian Physicians   69
7. Medical Officers' Assignments   76
8. Surgeons Afloat   92
9. Medical Purveying   108
10. Hospitals   123
11. Treating the Sick   140
12. Rendering Judgments   158
13. Sundry Activities   170
14. End and Aftermath of the War   178

Conclusion   182
Appendix A. Commissioned Medical Officers in the CSN   189
Appendix B. Duties of Medical Officers   195
Chapter Notes   199
Bibliography   221
Index   231

Foreword

BY GARY MCQUARRIE

When the Confederate capital of Richmond, Virginia, was evacuated on April 3, 1865, fires consumed much of the city. In addition to causing massive destruction, they deprived Civil War historians of a large number of documents and records that would have been very helpful in reconstructing and detailing a fuller history of the Confederate States Navy (CSN), including its medical services. The latter has remained an insufficiently researched area, with only limited efforts and published material at least partially addressing the subject in the last 60 years.

Published works about the Union and Confederate navies and their officers seem to be somewhat proportional to the size of the two navies, perhaps because a larger volume of Union historical records was preserved. Regardless, readership interest in the CSN and its exploits remains considerable, particularly among Southerners, in part as a point of naval pride. Given its considerable disadvantages, the CSN fielded formidable and feared warships, and it had its share of officers who demonstrated notable courage and daring in action. Civil War historians and those generally interested in the war's history tend to focus on the armies while ignoring or underemphasizing the relative roles and impact of *both navies* in the conflict and its course.

When the war broke out, the "old Navy" (the U.S. Navy, USN) had only 52 serviceable vessels, many on overseas stations, with the remainder lying in ordinary. To successfully implement its "Anaconda" plan of strangling the South by controlling its waterways and blockading its ports, hundreds of vessels would be built

Foreword

or purchased, with the USN eventually comprising more than 650 ships, including more than 25 monitors and 15 river ironclads.[1]

The Confederates had only a few state navies with a small number of ships to begin with. By early 1862, they began focusing most of their efforts on constructing ironclads that could defeat the Union's wooden ships on its rivers and along its coasts. In total, the South fielded approximately 130 warships (including about 25 ironclads) and perhaps more than 150 unarmed steamers and transports. The South was at a significant disadvantage in materials, machinery, workers, and shipbuilding facilities, and these deficits would prove pivotal. Notably, at New Orleans in April 1862, had the Confederate ironclads *Louisiana* and *Mississippi* been fully operational, the capture of the Crescent City by Flag Officer David G. Farragut's squadron of wooden ships might have been prevented. Instead, the Union gained control over the South's most important port and access to the lower Mississippi River, which altered the course of the war. Nonetheless, the CSN, particularly in its use of ironclads, compiled a record of ingenuity and bravery in battle despite overwhelming odds.[2]

The numbers of sailors and officers needed to crew the navies was essentially proportional to the size of each navy's combined fleet. Service in the USN was definitively safer than service in the U.S. Army, with the rate of combat deaths and casualties in the navy being about a fifth of that in the army. The U.S. Marines had slightly higher rates of combat deaths and casualties than sailors, probably because of their involvement in onshore engagements. Corresponding casualty rates, based on comparable data, for the Confederate navy and marine corps are not available, but there are no apparent reasons why they would differ significantly from those for Union forces. Substantial violence, however, did occur in naval engagements, with the majority of combat deaths and injuries occurring as a result of cannon fire from enemy warships or shore batteries. Occasionally, deaths or wounding resulted from gunshots, cutlasses, accidents, or scalding from steam.[3]

Importantly, disease—primarily malarial fevers, typhoid, yellow fever, and dysentery and diarrhea—significantly affected both navies'

Foreword

personnel, particularly on rivers and in marshy and coastal areas. In the Union navy and marine corps, causes other than combat resulted in fewer deaths than combat itself. On the Mississippi River in the summer of 1862, the functional capacities of Farragut's squadron and Flag Officer Charles H. Davis's Western Gunboat Flotilla were seriously degraded because large proportions of the crews were on the sick list. Similar disease impacts occurred in Confederate naval ranks along the Mississippi and in the squadrons on the James River and at Savannah and Mobile. In either navy, appropriate medical care was thus a critically important aspect of maintaining operational and fighting capabilities. The need to manage casualties and disease combined with the lack of accommodations on board individual vessels prompted the creation of the USN's first hospital ship, *Red Rover*, to care for sick or wounded sailors and also to be able to quickly transport patients to shore-based hospitals for care.[4]

Because of differences in the preservation of records and unofficial accounts, far more information and details are available on the medical services of the Union than the Confederate navy. The subject area generally seems to be of lesser interest to most Civil War readers and historians, compared with the medical services and care provided by both armies, perhaps in part because of the sheer scale of deaths and casualties that occurred in the land war. After recently researching and documenting the organization and services of the Confederate army's medical department,[5] Guy R. Hasegawa offers a new work, *The Confederate Navy Medical Corps: Organization, Personnel and Actions*, that addresses a relatively neglected area of the war's naval medical history, medical services for the CSN. Hasegawa is a clinically trained pharmacist by profession and spent more than 30 years as an editor for hospital pharmacy's premier professional journal. He is a meticulous researcher and well-published writer and speaker in the area of Civil War medicine. In this book, he details thoroughly the readily available information, such as official Confederate government reports and communications, physician diaries and medical data contained therein, medical officer registers, the few personal accounts of those serving in the naval medical corps, and selected compilations of data. Importantly, besides the traditional

Foreword

archival research of records held in libraries and special collections, this work is underpinned by close examination of relevant information available only on National Archives microfilm. This approach unearthed many previously unreported details and provided new insight into multiple aspects of the subject area.

In establishing a naval medical corps, the Confederacy generally followed USN traditions and overall organization and benefited by the resignations of USN medical officers who joined the Southern navy. Hasegawa describes these origins of the naval medical organization and services in depth and chronicles and explains how initial and ongoing Confederate congressional legislation helped to shape the organization and its personnel. This approach, often overlooked by historians, provides critical perspective on the course of developments. He also provides a comprehensive table full of details on all commissioned Confederate naval medical officers. This entire section of this book is particularly outstanding. But Hasegawa continues to describe in a similarly detailed, comprehensive, and logical manner every other aspect of providing naval medical services. These topics include physician evaluation, surgeons' stewards and hospital stewards, medical services afloat or in shore facilities, and illnesses encountered and medications utilized. The work also contains the most comprehensive bibliography on the subject compiled to date.

Hasegawa, in his conclusion, places his own work in clear perspective, noting gaps in records that could help complete the historical picture. Further advancing the subject may depend on unearthing heretofore undiscovered documents. *The Confederate Navy Medical Corps: Organization, Personnel and Actions* will be most welcome by readers interested in the Confederate navy and its medical services. Not only does it help to fill a gap in the historical literature, but it is also likely to become *the* reference source on the topic for many years to come.

Gary McQuarrie is the managing editor of Civil War Navy—The Magazine.

Preface

Although there is a fair amount of literature on medical care in the armies of the American Civil War, the medical activities of the navies have received little attention. This is especially true for the Confederate States Navy (CSN). Medical care in the CSN has been addressed in two short articles and briefly in books on the CSN—Tomblin's *Life in Jefferson Davis' Navy* is a recent example—but no in-depth exploration of the topic has been available. This void in the historical literature, which *The Confederate Navy Medical Corps: Organization, Personnel and Actions* aims to fill, has been unfortunate, because the navies played a vital role in the conduct of the war, and their operational efficiency was strongly related to the health of their personnel. Historians who had considered delving into Confederate naval medicine, it seems, had been discouraged by the scarcity of relevant period documents and the difficulty of using them.[1]

Most records kept at the Richmond headquarters of the CSN medical corps are thought to have been lost either in the fire that consumed large parts of the Confederate capital in April 1865 or during the flight of Confederate officials from the city. It was customary, however, for officers to keep copies of government correspondence, and some papers in the hands of naval personnel stationed throughout the South—including parts of Richmond that did not burn—survived the war and are available to researchers. Unfortunately, wartime diaries or personal journals of CSN medical officers are few, as are postwar reminiscences that deal with their medically related experiences.

Having spent much of my historical effort over the years to the study of medicine in the Civil War armies, I explored more than once the possibility of extending my research to the CSN. I started with

Preface

the naval *Official Records*, which contain three reports submitted by Surgeon William A.W. Spotswood, chief of the CSN medical department, to Stephen R. Mallory, the Confederate secretary of the navy. These authoritative and explanatory documents, along with additional correspondence in the naval *Official Records*, were vital but provided nothing more than what other authors had already summarized. It was clear that unpublished archival material had to be consulted, and my first attempt to do so, in the early 2000s, began with a key microfilm series—the Subject File of the Confederate States Navy (M1031)—at the National Archives and Records Administration (NARA) in Washington, D.C. At the time, I was primarily interested in pharmacy and medical purveying, and scrolling through the relevant film rolls was tedious and discouraging. Most documents pertained to the sale of goods or services to the CSN by various firms or individuals, but there was little to explain how those transactions fit into the big picture, whatever that might be. I concluded at least twice that I lacked the patience and background knowledge to continue. After all, thorough examination of the film would require multiple trips to NARA, and returning to potentially useful images would be time-consuming because the film does not have frame numbers.

That situation changed vastly when it became possible to view NARA microfilm M1031 and other CSN-relevant microfilm online. The microfilmed documents, most of which are handwritten, have not been converted to a form amenable to full-text searching, yet the material's easy and convenient accessibility and the ability to return quickly to images of interest greatly facilitated research and, frankly, made this book possible. Various period publications that had been hard to locate and consult also because viewable online over the years, a development that again saved much time and effort. Expanding my research beyond medical purveying resulted from having source documents in easier-to-use form and from my realization that understanding purveying required an appreciation of how the entire medical department operated.

The nature of available documents dictated that this book focus on the organizational aspects of CSN medicine. Because official

Preface

documents are much more common than personal accounts of medical service, it is easier to describe what, and occasionally why, medical personnel did rather than what they thought about it. The book is arranged thematically to facilitate the understanding of various actions and decisions and to help readers interpret information that becomes available in the future. To do otherwise—to present all events in strict chronological sequence, for example—would have required frequent explanatory but distracting tangents. The thematic approach, though, necessitates some redundancy, because a specific incident was often the result of multiple concurrent influences or because it might illustrate more than one concept. Readers who wish to place the actions of the medical department into the larger context of what the entire navy was doing should consult one of the fine general histories of the CSN.

This book is by no means a complete account of CSN medicine; indeed, many questions remain unanswered. Gaps in the historical record, for example, make it hard to characterize the nature of medical services west of the Mississippi River and throughout the Confederacy in the final months of the war. I have, though, tried to make this book as comprehensive as the available sources allow while avoiding minutiae that would add little to understanding. My hope is that it fills a gap in the literature, becomes a useful reference, and serves as a springboard for future research. *The Confederate Navy Medical Corps: Organization, Personnel and Actions* is thoroughly documented, which should save time for readers wishing to verify, expand on, or even challenge my findings.

Research for this book spanned the most devastating periods of the Covid-19 pandemic, during which many libraries and other repositories were closed to researchers. I am grateful to the numerous individuals who assisted me by sending scans of documents from their institutions' collections. Among them were Megan Casey, Supervisory Librarian of the Reference Section, and Heidrun Perez, Technical Information Specialist, at the Navy Department Library, Naval History and Heritage Command, Washington, D.C., who cheerfully sent me scans from the library's collection of ZB (personnel) files. Jeffery Seymour, Director of History and Collections,

Preface

National Civil War Naval Museum, Columbus, Georgia, provided a transcript of the very useful diary of Dr. Robert Reeve Gibbes. Valuable assistance was also provided by numerous individuals at NARA, the Library of Congress, and many other repositories.

Expert assistance was provided by F. Terry Hambrecht, MD; Jonathan O'Neal, MD; and Gary McQuarrie, PharmD, MBA. All three read the manuscript and offered valuable suggestions for improvement. Terry, an authority on Civil War medicine, provided biographical summaries of CSN surgeons from an unpublished register—maintained by himself and Jodi Koste of Virginia Commonwealth University—of physicians who served the Confederacy in a medical capacity. Jonathan, another expert on Civil War medicine, offered the use of images from his collection. Gary, managing editor of *Civil War Navy—The Magazine*, honored me by contributing this book's foreword.

I am grateful to McFarland and editor Elizabeth Foxwell for seeing the value in this project and seeing it through the publication process.

My endeavors in Civil War medicine have always been supported by my wife, Betsy, and our sons, David and Stephen. This book is dedicated to them.

Introduction

As Southern lawmakers in Montgomery, Alabama, began forming the government of the new Confederate States of America in February 1861, the probable scope of any upcoming armed conflict with the North was unclear, as was the role that a Confederate navy might play. By February 2, seven Southern states had seceded in response to the November 1860 election of Abraham Lincoln as the next president of the United States; some had seized Federal military assets within their borders or begun to form their own naval forces.[1]

It was in that setting that the Committee on Naval Affairs of the new Provisional Confederate Congress invited in mid–February 1861 a number of naval experts to Montgomery to advise it on organizing a navy. After consulting the advisors, the committee concluded that "any very extensive naval preparations in time to meet the dangers that threaten us are impracticable." Indeed, the South had no important vessels and had only one navy yard, the former U.S. Navy (USN) facility near Pensacola, Florida, which had been seized by Alabama and Florida state troops in mid–January.[2]

With those limitations in mind, the Provisional Congress proceeded to create the Confederate States Navy (CSN) in an act approved by new Confederate president Jefferson Davis on February 21, 1861. The Navy Department would be administered by the secretary of the navy, who would act under the direction and control of the president. Davis's choice for the naval secretary was Stephen R. Mallory, a former U.S. senator from Florida who had resigned his seat on January 21, 1861. Mallory, whose service in the U.S. Senate started in 1851, had a special interest in naval matters and had served on the Committee on Naval Affairs from late 1851 until his resignation from the Senate; for about half of that time—starting in late

Introduction

1855—he had chaired that committee. After some debate, the Provisional Congress on March 4, 1861, confirmed Mallory's appointment as secretary of the Navy Department. Mallory served in that capacity throughout the war.[3]

Among the many immediate decisions faced by Mallory were how to organize his department and whom to appoint to head its major divisions. Of no small importance was seeing to the health of the men who would make up the navy. Mallory knew that the general efficiency of his navy would depend on its health but also that major outbreaks of disease could seriously impair the navy's fighting strength. Furthermore, if the public were to believe that the navy provided poor health services, recruitment of new personnel—in which the navy lagged behind the army—would suffer.

By late in the war, the CSN contained on its rolls about 4,500 enlisted men and 750 officers, who would depend on medical officers to treat their illnesses and injuries and help maintain their health. Naval surgeons would also be tending to members of the Confederate States Marine Corps, eventually numbering more than 500. Medical officers would not only be assigned to duty afloat—if and when the navy succeeded in procuring vessels of war—they would also be needed at shore facilities, such as hospitals and navy yards. An adequate number of competent medical officers would have to be appointed, and enlisted men would have to be found to assist those officers. Although the scale of naval combat could not be anticipated, Southern physicians could probably predict that malaria and other illnesses would be common in sailors and marines spending much of their time in coastal areas. Shore-based hospitals would have to be located where large numbers of naval personnel were stationed, especially in the event of a prolonged or large-scale war. Since the prewar South was not producing substantial quantities of medical goods, the curtailment of trade with the North and the imposition of a naval blockade portended trouble in obtaining sufficient supplies for the treatment of sailors and marines. Medical staffing of vessels and shore facilities would have to be flexible enough to adapt to adjustments in naval strategy and wartime developments.[4]

To some extent, the CSN's medical corps could model its orga-

Introduction

nization after its Union counterpart. The CSN could also begin with men of experience, since many USN officers of Southern origin, including surgeons, resigned their commissions to join the Confederate cause. Nevertheless, the CSN was destined to get a slow start. In February 1862, about a year after the Provisional Confederate Congress established the Navy Department, President Davis described the CSN's early difficulties: "The people of the Confederate States, being principally engaged in agricultural pursuits, were unprovided at the commencement of hostilities with ships, ship-yards, materials for ship-building, or skilled mechanics and seamen in sufficient numbers to make the prompt creation of a navy a practicable task."[5]

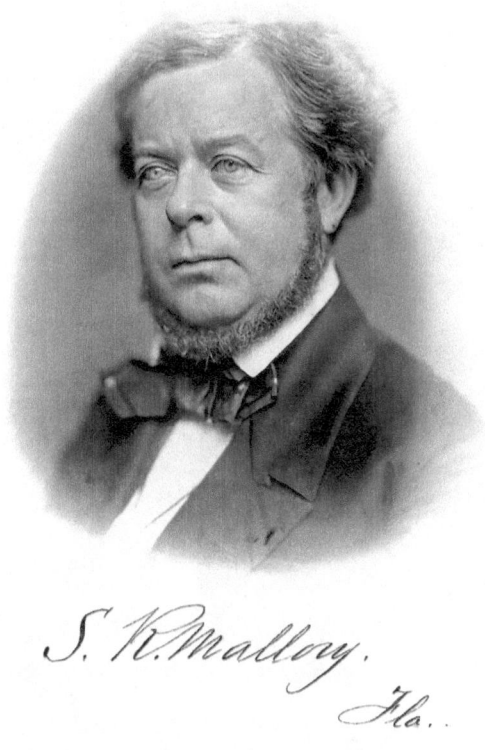

Stephen R. Mallory as a U.S. senator from Florida ca. 1859. Mallory served throughout the Civil War as Confederate secretary of the navy (James E. McClees and Julian Vannerson, *McClees' Gallery of Photographic Portraits of the Senators, Representatives & Delegates of the Thirty-Fifth Congress* [Washington, D.C.: McClees and Beck, (1859?)]. Library of Congress, control no. 2010649422).

Thus, the CSN and its medical department faced substantial challenges from the start. How those challenges were met by the department's leadership and by its commissioned, enlisted, and civilian personnel is chronicled and detailed in this work.

– 1 –

Beginnings of the Medical Corps

As an expedient in forming the Confederate government, the Provisional Congress adopted all U.S. laws not in conflict with the new Confederate constitution. In fact, many Confederate government entities, such as the army, patterned their organization and practices after their U.S. counterparts. Thus, it is no surprise that when the general structure of the CSN was set forth in an act of March 16, 1861, it resembled that of the USN. That legislation created divisions, as yet unnamed, within the CSN that came to be known as the Office of Orders and Detail, Office of Ordnance and Hydrography, Office of Provisions and Clothing, and Office of Medicine and Surgery (OMS); additional offices were authorized by later legislation. The divisions partially replicated those used by the USN since 1842: the Bureau of Yards and Docks; Bureau of Construction, Equipment and Repair; Bureau of Ordnance and Hydrography; Bureau of Provisions and Clothing; and Bureau of Medicine and Surgery. The USN's bureau chiefs were appointed by the president with Senate approval, whereas the Confederate act of March 16 was silent on how the chiefs of the various CSN offices were to be appointed; in fact, they were named by Secretary Mallory. The CSN office chiefs were each allowed a clerk but would receive no compensation beyond their regular pay.[1]

Whereas the USN's Bureau of Medicine and Surgery was directed by a full surgeon, the CSN's OMS was to be headed by a surgeon or assistant surgeon who, under the direction of the secretary of the navy, was to "make all purchases of medicines and medical supplies for the navy, and perform such other duties appertaining to the medical department as the secretary may from time to time direct." (Although *surgeon* could refer generically to any military physician, whether he performed surgical procedures or not, it was also a naval grade that was superior to various grades of assistant surgeon. In this book, the term *full surgeon* appears when needed to distinguish among grades of medical officers.) That job description suggests that, in light of the modest force being formed, Confederate legislators believed that there would be little more to minding the health of the navy than ensuring that it had adequate medical supplies. Regardless of what Mallory thought at the time, he would surely come to expect more from the OMS chief.[2]

During Mallory's chairmanship of the U.S. Senate Committee on Naval Affairs, the second edition of official instructions for USN medical officers was issued. It stated that the chief of the Bureau of Medicine and Surgery was responsible for "general supervision and control of every thing relating to the treatment of the sick and wounded of the Navy." Furthermore, the chief would "keep a record of the services of medical officers, and nominate them for duty" and receive and forward "all official communications from medical officers" intended for the Navy Department. Mallory may have known that when the USN's Bureau of Medicine and Surgery was first formed, Secretary of the Navy Abel P. Upshur declared that the bureau chief "ought to be, and it is presumed always will be, a man of a high order of professional attainments and general education, holding a social position equal in all respects, to that of any other man."[3]

During Mallory's term in the U.S. Senate, the Bureau of Medicine and Surgery was under its second and third chiefs. The first, Surgeon William P.C. Barton, stood second in seniority among USN medical officers when appointed to that position in 1842. The officer senior to him, Jonathan Cowdery, may have been passed over because he was then 75 years old (Barton was almost 56) and had not been particularly active for some time. Barton resigned as bureau chief and was replaced in 1844 by Thomas Harris, third on the list of surgeons below Cowdery and Barton. When Harris left that position in 1853, the nomination of Surgeon William Whelan to replace him

1. Beginnings of the Medical Corps

was confirmed on the recommendation of the Committee on Naval Affairs, which included Mallory.[4]

Thus, Mallory was familiar with the extensive duties of the chief of the Bureau of Medicine and Surgery and was probably well aware that the first two appointees had been—after the exclusion of Cowdery—the most senior surgeons in the navy. It is notable that Whelan stood 25th among 69 surgeons in seniority when he became bureau chief, yet he still boasted 25 years of naval service when appointed. Mallory's background, plus his observation of the creditable service of Harris and Whelan, should have given him a good idea of the type of officer who should lead the CSN's OMS, especially if the CSN were destined for substantial growth.[5]

Mallory probably envisioned the eventual responsibilities of the OMS chief as extending beyond purchasing supplies to overall direction of the medical corps. Such an assignment could certainly not go to an assistant surgeon but must be filled by a full surgeon with a respectable amount of seniority. Furthermore, if the OMS chief were an assistant surgeon, he would be issuing orders to—and be paid less than—some officers who had much more naval service, and that was a scenario bound to cause friction. On March 12, 1861, four days before legislation organizing the CSN was approved, Mallory recorded a cost estimate that assumed that the OMS chief would receive the salary of a full surgeon with at least 10 years at that grade.

Exactly when Mallory chose the OMS chief is unclear, but among the naval medical officers available to the Confederacy before mid–June 1861, Surgeon William A.W. Spotswood had the most seniority and received the appointment. Spotswood served in that role throughout most of the war, despite the fact that by mid–September 1861, two medical officers who had been senior to him in the USN, James Cornick and William F. Patton, had entered the CSN. By November 1, 1862, the charge of the OMS chief was formally expanded to duplicate that of his USN counterpart: "general supervision and control of every thing relating to the treatment of the sick and wounded of the Navy," recording the services of medical officers, forwarding official communications from medical officers to

15

the Navy Department, and approving all requisitions and bills for medical supplies.⁶

Spotswood and the OMS

William Augustine Washington Spotswood was born in 1806 in Virginia into a family prominent in the commonwealth's history. He was a great-grandnephew of George Washington and a great-great-grandson of Alexander Spotswood, the colonial lieutenant governor of Virginia. Spotswood took medical and other courses at the University of Virginia, although it is unclear whether he ever received a medical degree. He entered the USN as an assistant surgeon in 1828 and was promoted to surgeon in 1838. His final cruise in the USN was as fleet surgeon with the East India Squadron, after which he was assigned to the Pensacola Naval Hospital in June 1860. Florida seceded from the Union on January 10, 1861, and two days later the Pensacola Navy Yard was seized by Alabama and Florida state troops. Spotswood then tendered his resignation from the USN on January 19, 1861, "by reason of the action of Florida in regard to the separation of the Southern States from the Federal Union." In resigning, said Spotswood, he "acted upon a principle which patriotism, conscience, and conviction to my duty to my native land prompted me to act, even while regretting and deploring the steps the Southern people were compelled to take, to vindicate their rights guaranteed by the Constitution." Spotswood entered the CSN as a surgeon on March 26, 1861, and evidently stayed at Pensacola—where he was paid by the CSN for the period of March 29 through April 30—until at least May 8.⁷

At some point early in the war, Spotswood moved all or part of his family from Pensacola to Monroeville, Alabama. Family matters, in fact, probably weighed heavily on Spotswood during the war. In September 1861, he appealed to Albert T. Bledsoe, chief of the War Department's administrative office, to consider Spotswood's oldest son, George Willis Spotswood, for a clerical position. George had previously worked at the CSN installation at Fort Barrancas, near

1. Beginnings of the Medical Corps

Pensacola, until the clerical force there was reduced and was "very anxious to go in the ranks as a volunteer." Because of his young age (about 18 years), George's mother wanted him to defer such service until the "exigencies of the country demanded every boy and man from the age of 16 to 70 years." George did subsequently work as a Navy Department clerk, but that was after he served for several months in the 2nd Florida Infantry Regiment. The Spotswoods' second son, Thomas Eastin Spotswood, enlisted in the 53rd Alabama Partisan Rangers and was captured at Resaca, Georgia, in May 1864, before he turned 17. He was imprisoned and eventually exchanged in March 1865. In March 1862, Surgeon Spotswood's wife, Mary Eastin Spotswood, give birth in Florida to another son, Dillon Jordan Spotswood.[8]

Surgeon Spotswood even spoke up to help a distant relative. Mary G. Spotswood of Virginia, a second cousin, once removed, of Surgeon Spotswood, started seeking a government clerical job by February 1864. When she applied again in October 1864, this time to Adjutant and Inspector General Samuel Cooper of the army, Surgeon Spotswood added an endorsement: "Miss Mary Spotswood is ... more needy than many who have been given appointments. The Yankees have destroyed everything in the house of her Father, who is an old man. She had 3 brothers [actually four] in the army. One has died from ill treatment by the Yankees, one now perhaps dying at home after having served 3 years—2 others still in the army—every vestage [sic] of property household furniture money negroes & clothes all gone. Do my dear Sir give her a place if possible." A clerical spot was found for Mary in the War Department.[9]

It has not been determined whether Surgeon Spotswood reported to the Navy Department at Montgomery or first took his place as the OMS chief after the capital was moved to Richmond in early June. In any event, the OMS had a presence in Montgomery, where Surgeon William F. Carrington took delivery of surgical instruments that were purchased in New Orleans on May 3, 1861, and purchased instruments himself in Montgomery on May 23, 1861. Some business relevant to the OMS was actually conducted before the Navy Department's offices were formally established on March 16. On March 12,

The Confederate Navy Medical Corps

Secretary Mallory prepared cost estimates for the only substantial facilities then in possession of the CSN, the Pensacola Navy Yard and Naval Hospital. Mallory also submitted, on April 26, 1861, a cost estimate for medical supplies for the year ending February 18, 1862. The predicted size of the navy was evident in Mallory's projection that surgical instruments and a medicine chest for each vessel—Mallory guessed there would be 10 such vessels—hospital, and receiving ship would total only $5,500. Supplies for the Pensacola Navy Yard, listed separately, were projected to cost $500.[10]

The Navy Department's first home in Richmond, shared with other departments and occupied for about a month, was the Custom House (also called the Treasury Building) on Bank Street. Around July 1, 1861, the War, Navy, and other departments moved to the Virginia Mechanics Institute building on Ninth Street between Main and Franklin Streets. The spacious structure, with some 50 rooms, was at the terminus of Bank Street and faced the southwest corner of Capitol Square. Secretary Mallory's office was on the second story—up the stairs from the ground floor—connected with spaces assigned to the chiefs of the navy's subordinate bureaus or offices. The OMS appears to have initially occupied space on the fourth story before moving to the second. One of the offices near Spotswood's was used by Thomas Cooper De Leon, chief clerk of the CSN's Office of Provisions and Clothing and brother of Surgeon David Camden De Leon, the first acting surgeon general of the Confederate army. Writing after the war, T.C. De Leon described Spotswood: "Towering high above average men, with muscular and vigorous frame, he walked with the roll of a veteran sailor; his long white beard bannered to the breeze." Another former Navy Department clerk said Spotswood was "a brawny, gray haired six-footer, rough and ready in ways and looks, but a gentle hearted man." No photograph of Spotswood has been found.[11]

Spotswood's one opening for a civilian clerk was filled by Francis Doyle and later by Charles N. Fennell. The latter, from Pensacola, had a teenaged son, Robert, who worked for the OMS as a messenger. In November 1864, Spotswood asked that a full surgeon be assigned to the OMS to help him in "directing and controlling the affairs of

1. Beginnings of the Medical Corps

the Medical Department." At the time, such assistance was mostly being provided by "newly appointed assistant surgeons." CSN registers through mid–1864 and other records beyond that point do not indicate medical officers other than Spotswood being assigned to the OMS. Whatever the size of the OMS staff, it was certainly dwarfed by that of its army counterpart, the Surgeon General's Office. There, also in November 1864, the staff numbered 35, including Surgeon General Samuel Preston Moore and five other surgeons, 11 enlisted men detailed for clerical work, and 18 civilian clerks (eight men and 10 women).[12]

Although Spotswood traveled from Richmond to Pensacola in September 1861, how often he was otherwise absent from the OMS is not known. It is clear, though, that direction of the office was put in other hands from time to time. Approving expenses incurred by medical officers was Spotswood's responsibility as the OMS chief, but Surgeon William B. Sinclair approved a voucher in December 1861, calling himself "Surgeon in Charge." On a voucher dated October, 24, 1862, Surgeon Richard W. Jeffery wrote "In charge of Med & Surgery Pro tem" under his approval signature, and on November 1, 1862, Jeffery was ordered to assume temporary charge of the OMS "in place of Surgeon Spotswood, who has been placed on leave of absence for a time." During the following few months, Jeffery affixed variations of "Surgeon in charge of office of Medicine & Surgery Navy Department" under his approval signature.[13]

Surgeon James F. Harrison, who directed the CSN hospital in Richmond, appears to have filled in for Spotswood most often. His name, with the title "Surgeon in Charge" of the Navy Department's OMS, accompanied that of the army surgeon general, Samuel Preston Moore, as endorsing a December 1863 petition of dental surgeons for exemption from military service. Harrison signed as being "in charge" in December 1863 and January 1864 for expenses incurred in North Carolina, and in late September 1864, he approved a voucher and identified himself as "in charge, Office Med. & Surgery, Temp'y."[14]

Although vouchers typically bore the date or dates on which expenses were incurred, approval signatures were usually undated

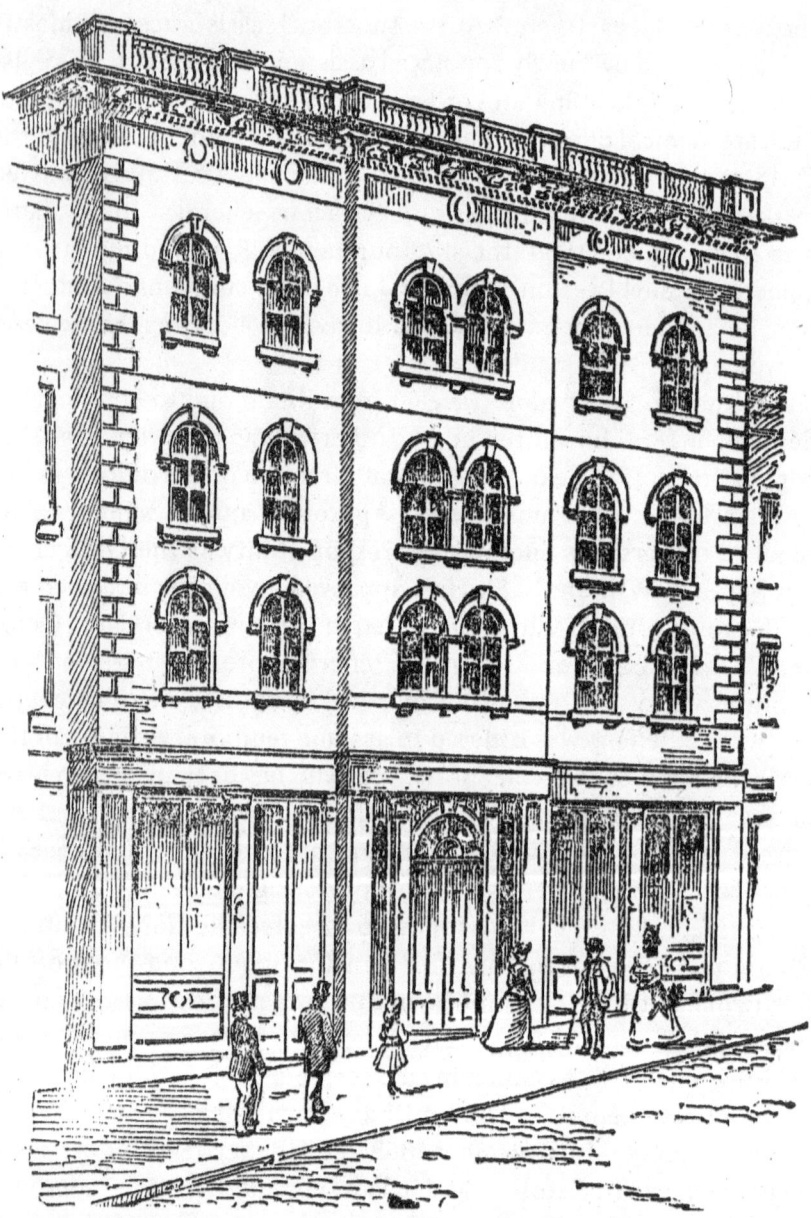

The Virginia Mechanics Institute building in Richmond, which housed the Confederate Navy and War department offices on its second story. The structure, built in 1858, was destroyed in the fire of April 1865 (*Richmond Dispatch*, June 30, 1896).

1. Beginnings of the Medical Corps

and could have been affixed months later. Spotswood approved vouchers that bore similar dates to those approved by Sinclair, Jeffery, and Harrison, but the absence of approval dates makes it impossible to determine exactly when Spotswood was unavailable. Jeffery's and Harrison's temporary OMS duties extended beyond approving vouchers. Official OMS estimates of costs submitted to Secretary Mallory were signed on December 16, 1862, by Jeffery (as "Surgeon Temporarily in Charge" of the OMS) and by Harrison on February 22, 1865 (as "in charge" of the OMS). Spotswood left Richmond on or about January 23, 1865, on leave of absence and did not return to duty during the remainder of the war. Harrison likely filled in for him during that time.[15]

Of course, Spotswood did much more than prepare budgets and approve expenses. He undoubtedly assisted Secretary Mallory in adapting USN regulations into a version, dated April 29, 1862, to be used by the CSN. The section of the CSN regulations describing the duties of medical officers was reprinted in a booklet, also adapted from a USN document, that was dated November 1, 1862: *Instructions for the Guidance of the Medical Officers of the Navy of the Confederate States*. The instructions also described the medicines and other supplies, and the amounts thereof, allowed per 100 men per year; multiple forms to be completed and submitted to the OMS; and medical terms to be used when describing disease and injury. All of these features appeared in the USN instructions, but Spotswood had to adapt them to the needs of the CSN.[16]

In an effort to share knowledge and encourage camaraderie among the Confederacy's medical officers, the army surgeon general, Samuel Preston Moore, prompted the formation of the Association of Army and Navy Surgeons of the Confederate States (AANS), which was to meet every two weeks at the Medical College of Virginia (MCV) in Richmond. Membership was open to all army and naval surgeons. At the organization's first session on August 22, 1863, Moore was elected president, and Surgeon Spotswood was elected one of the vice presidents. At the September 5, 1863, meeting, however, Spotswood's resignation as vice president was received and accepted; his reason for resigning was not recorded. Spotswood's position appears to have been filled by Surgeon Daniel B. Conrad, CSN.[17]

In January 1864, Richmond publishers Ayres and Wade released the first issue of the *Confederate States Medical and Surgical Journal*, which was intended to inform readers of AANS activities, publish interesting case reports, share important statistics and trends in Confederate medicine, and provide recent knowledge from European medical journals. Although Spotswood did not contribute to the new publication, Surgeon Richard W. Jeffery—who had filled in for Spotswood at the OMS on more than one occasion—wrote a case report for the March 1864 issue. Jeffery, then stationed at the Savannah Naval Hospital, described a seaman of Confederate States ship (CSS) *Isondiga* who had received a fatal gunshot wound to the chest while visiting a brothel. It has not been determined how many CSN medical officers were AANS members or subscribed to the journal—both required fees—but it seems likely that Surgeon Spotswood would have encouraged both.[18]

Only the Start

The initial charge of the OMS—to purchase medical supplies—was challenge enough, given the South's relative lack of an industrial base (including those producing medical stores), the Union naval blockade, and competition among aggressive buyers for goods already in merchants' hands or arriving via blockade-running. Specific efforts, then, would be needed to ensure a reliable supply chain. Sick or injured sailors at sea were often treated aboard, but more serious cases or those occurring in shore facilities might require hospitals, which had to be established, staffed, and supervised.

The reports that Surgeon Spotswood submitted to Secretary Mallory give some indication of the OMS's other concerns. Spotswood, for example, tracked the number of officers he had of each grade, their assignments, and whether their numbers were adequate for the CSN's activities. He described the general health of the navy, presented statistics on hospitalizations and deaths, and

1. Beginnings of the Medical Corps

recommended changes that might reduce sickness. He tried to protect his civilian employees from being taken for army service or replaced by persons with no relevant expertise, and he praised the dedication and efficiency of his medical officers. He described the department's expenses and projected funding needs. Spotswood could not have prepared detailed reports without collecting and analyzing masses of paperwork from the numerous vessels and shore installations where his officers were stationed.[19]

Clearly, Spotswood would have to organize the OMS into an efficient operation. The tasks he eventually performed—and the mission of the medical corps in seeing to the health of the navy—could not be accomplished without the necessary personnel.

– 2 –

Building a Nucleus

It was recognized early that former USN officers would form the nucleus of the CSN. On February 13, 1861, the Provisional Confederate Congress agreed "that the Committee on Military Affairs [for the army] and the Committee on Naval Affairs be instructed to include in any plan they may propose for the organization of the Army and Navy, suitable provision for such officers of the Army and Navy of the United States as may have tendered a resignation of their commissions in consequence of their adhesion to any or all of the States of this Confederacy." Such officers would include those who had entered state navies—which were absorbed into the CSN—and those who had not.[1]

Given the CSN's slow start, its initial size and complexity were necessarily limited. The March 16, 1861, legislation that first organized the CSN allowed for the appointment of only five surgeons and five assistant surgeons; those openings would presumably include the officer chosen to head the OMS. The grade of passed assistant surgeon, which existed in the USN, was omitted. (Passed assistant surgeons were assistant surgeons who had passed the examination qualifying them for promotion to surgeon and were waiting for a vacancy in the roll of surgeons through death, resignation, or dismissal.) Although the March 16 legislation did not so state, it was expected that positions for officers would be filled by men who had resigned from the USN as a consequence of Southern secession. By April 20, 1861, one surgeon slot was filled by Spotswood, the only available former USN officer of that grade, and the other four went to former Passed Assistant Surgeons William F. Carrington, Francis L. Galt, Arthur M. Lynah, and John Ward. (Because the grade of CSN passed assistant surgeon did not then exist, former USN officers of that grade entered the CSN as surgeons.) By the same date, only two of the five slots for assistant surgeons were filled, by former USN Assistant Surgeons Charles E. Lining and Thomas J. Charlton, Jr.[2]

Leaving the USN

Filling the openings for CSN surgeons and assistant surgeons depended on current USN medical officers leaving their positions. In fact, among medical officers who would enter the CSN, the first resignation from the USN came even before the end of 1860. The aforementioned Thomas J. Charlton, Jr., a Georgia native and assistant surgeon in the USN, tendered his resignation on December 14, 1860, six days before the December 20 secession of South Carolina. After his resignation was accepted by the USN, Charlton was commissioned into the newly formed navy of Georgia as an assistant surgeon on February 1, 1861, and then began serving in the CSN in April 1861 at the same grade.[3]

Charlton received a CSN commission despite resigning from the USN before, rather than as a consequence of, secession. In at least two instances, former USN medical officers were excluded from appointment in the CSN because their resignations were much earlier than Charlton's. The first example was Wyatt M. Brown of North Carolina, who entered the USN as an assistant surgeon in 1854 and resigned in 1858. He applied for a position in the CSN in February 1861 and reported that Secretary Mallory indicated on May 1, 1861, that "no appointments were being made in his Department outside of those officers who have recently resigned." Brown subsequently received an appointment in the North Carolina navy and was later commissioned as an army surgeon for a North Carolina infantry regiment. Mallory's decision in Brown's case may have reflected his advance knowledge of an act that would be approved on May 20, 1861, which would allow the president to appoint to the CSN, with congressional approval, all former USN officers—regardless of number—who were fit for active service and had resigned because of secession. Secretary Mallory was unambiguous in his interpretation that the new law excluded any other applicants from appointment as CSN officers.[4]

The second example was Alexander Y.P. Garnett, who had served as an assistant surgeon in the USN from 1841 until his resignation in 1850. He moved from Washington, D.C., to Richmond in May 1861 and was appointed as assistant, at the grade of surgeon, in the Navy of Virginia's Bureau of Medicine and Surgery. Because Garnett's early resignation made him ineligible for appointment as a CSN officer, he asked the Provisional Confederate Congress to make an exception in his case. That evidently did not happen, and Garnett accepted a commission as surgeon in the Confederate army. The act of May 20—or Mallory's interpretation of it—thus deprived the CSN of at least two physicians with substantial military practice experience.[5]

It was not unusual for a handful of USN medical officers to resign during a year. In 1855 through 1859, for example, an average of four such officers, out of about 149, resigned per year. In 1861, however, 36 surgeons, passed assistant surgeons, or assistant surgeons tendered their resignation. Most, but not all, of those 36 were from the South and subsequently received a commission to serve in the CSN pursuant to the act of May 20, 1861, which removed the initial allowance (set by the act of March 16) of five surgeons and five assistant surgeons. Half of those tendered resignations occurred during May 1861.[6]

During the few months before the Civil War began, Isaac Toucey, the U.S. secretary of the navy under President James Buchanan, accepted all resignations tendered by officers of Southern origin in a routine procedure amounting to an honorable discharge. That practice generally continued from the early weeks of the Lincoln administration, which began in March 1861, until the early part of May 1861, when resignations submitted by officers from Southern states tended to result in those men being dismissed from the service by order of the president. Such dismissal was evidently intended to confer shame—"not a pleasant thing," according to one Southerner, "for their descendants to contemplate"—and was considered by CSN officers to be a spiteful policy of the Lincoln administration. Another

2. Building a Nucleus

Lincoln policy was to require current U.S. officers to reaffirm their oath of loyalty to the United States.[7]

Officers often believed themselves forced to resign by circumstances. Passed Assistant Surgeon Charles H. Williamson from Virginia described his regret at leaving the USN: "No one more deplored the unfortunate course of events that brought on the war than I, no one was more devotedly attached to the Union, and no one left a service in which I had spent many years with greater reluctance, but I had to yield in the struggle between duty to the government and devotion to my home."[8]

The decision to leave the USN could be prolonged. Surgeon William D. Harrison of Virginia, on duty aboard a USN vessel when the war began, recognized the powerful factors at play: "My entire family, with two exceptions, my relations, friends and interests of every description were, and have always been, in the South." His ship was ordered home in August 1861, and although he had been away from American soil for two years and wanted desperately to see his family, he put off resigning from the USN by volunteering to transfer to another vessel just beginning a cruise. The delay was of no benefit, for his "expectation, however, of a speedy termination of the difficulties between the [Northern and Southern] sections" was disappointed. His tendered resignation resulted, on February 3, 1863, in dismissal. Harrison entered the CSN on March 6, 1863, he explained, "to provide for those who were unchangeably fixed in that part of the country [the South]—And I do not believe that human nature could have acted very differently under the circumstances."[9]

At least two men commissioned as surgeons in the CSN, James W.B. Greenhow and James Cornick, had been placed on the USN's "retired list"—Greenhow on May 14 and Cornick on June 18, 1861—shortly before they tendered their resignations from the USN. U.S. legislation enacted in February 1861 authorized the president "to place on a retired list any medical officer of the navy who is now or may hereafter be proved to be permanently incapable, from physical or mental infirmity, of further service at sea." Medical officers so designated would be removed from active service, command, and line of promotion while receiving leave-of-absence pay. It has not been determined whether the two officers' placement on the retired list influenced their decisions to resign from the USN or was known by OMS chief Spotswood or Secretary Mallory. In any event, both medical officers served in the CSN throughout the war, with Cornick's assignments apparently limited to shore duty. Greenhow's CSN service included duty afloat, including an interval as a fleet surgeon.[10]

Notifying the U.S. Navy Department of one's desire to resign could result in consequences beyond dismissal. Surgeon Richard W. Jeffery (from Virginia), Passed Assistant Surgeon William M. Page (from Virginia), and Assistant Surgeon James E. Lindsay (from North Carolina) were at sea with the USN's Africa Squadron when they submitted letters of resignation in mid–July 1861. Jeffery's resignation was especially poignant: "No official act of my life has even been performed with as much pain; but believing it due to myself & to the service, it must be done, though it removes me from associations of a most happy character & from many of my most cherished friends." Letters of dismissal for Jeffery, Page, and Lindsay, issued in late September and early October 1861, were to take effect when received, but it is unclear whether they reached their addressees before those officers returned to the United States. Jeffery reported being arrested in Philadelphia in October, and by middle of that month, all three found themselves imprisoned at Fort Warren in Boston Harbor because, according to a former prisoner there, they had refused to take the loyalty oath. Jeffery, Page, and Lindsay were exchanged in late January 1862 for Union surgeons held prisoner in Richmond and later entered the CSN.[11]

The Act of May 20 in Operation

As a consequence of the act of May 20, 1861, which removed the original limits of five surgeons and five assistant surgeons, the CSN medical corps contained 21 surgeons and 12 assistant surgeons by the end of 1861. The full surgeons included 13 former USN surgeons and eight former USN passed assistant surgeons. Among the 33 men entering the CSN as medical officers before 1862, most (20) had been

2. Building a Nucleus

born in Virginia, followed by Georgia (four), Maryland and South Carolina (three each), North Carolina (two), and Arkansas (one). The Virginia predominance was more obvious among men appointed as surgeon (16 of 21) than assistant surgeon (four of 12).[12]

Despite Secretary Mallory's belief that the May 20 act restricted appointments to former USN officers, three new CSN assistant surgeons—Theodosius Bartow Ford, Robert R. Gibbes, and Charles M. Morfit—had little or no service in the USN. How President Davis came to nominate Ford, a physician from Georgian, is unclear. On May 11, 1861, Ford enlisted as a private in a Georgia infantry regiment. A week later, newspapers announced his appointment as an assistant surgeon in the CSN, and on May 21, he was nominated and confirmed for that role.[13]

Gibbes (in 1860) and Morfit (in 1861) had applied to become USN assistant surgeons and performed satisfactorily when examined by a naval medical board. Records documenting Gibbes's appointment to or service in the USN have not been found, yet he described in his diary having entered Federal service. Morfit, a Marylander, was sent a letter of appointment as assistant surgeon, USN, on May 9, 1861, but the appointment was revoked several days later. He received an appointment in May 1861 as assistant surgeon in the Navy of Virginia, an organization that recruited Virginians or Virginia residents who had recently resigned from the USN. When the CSN accepted officers from the Virginia navy, it took Morfit to be a former USN assistant surgeon from Virginia, although he was neither. Those assumptions were later corrected—the 1863 and 1864 CSN registers of officers showed Morfit as a Marylander lacking previous USN service—without apparent consequences to Morfit. The CSN may have welcomed Gibbes and Morfit because they had recently passed the rigid entrance requirements for new USN assistant surgeons.[14]

State Navies as Sources of Medical Officers

The eagerness of some physicians to enter military service prompted them to seek positions with state navies, which were later

The Confederate Navy Medical Corps

absorbed into the CSN. Virginia invited "all efficient and worthy Virginians and residents of Virginia" who were in the U.S. military—apparently including non–Virginians assigned to duty in Virginia—to resign and enter the state's army or navy at a rank at least equivalent to that held in Federal service. Of the state navies, Virginia's provided the largest number of medical officers by far (16) to the CSN. They included (with grade in the Virginia navy shown) Surgeons George Blacknall, James F. Harrison, John T. Mason, Randolph F. Mason, William F. McClenahan, Lewis W. Minor, William F. Patton, and William B. Sinclair; Passed Assistant Surgeons Daniel B. Conrad, Dinwiddie B. Phillips, Henry W.M. Washington, Charles H. Williamson, and William E. Wysham; and Assistant Surgeons Bennett W. Green, Charles M. Morfit, and Frederic Van Bibber (later known as Frederic Garretson). All of those officers entered the CSN in June 1861. (Other former USN officers from Virginia entered the CSN before or after the existence of the Virginia navy.) One former USN medical officer, Morris B. Beck, served briefly in Virginia's navy but was denied a commission in that organization because he was thought to lack the prerequisite of being "efficient." Beck had entered the USN in 1841, was declared in 1853 by a medical survey to be "incapable of duty," and resigned as a passed assistant surgeon on May 10, 1861. The yearly USN registers for 1854–61

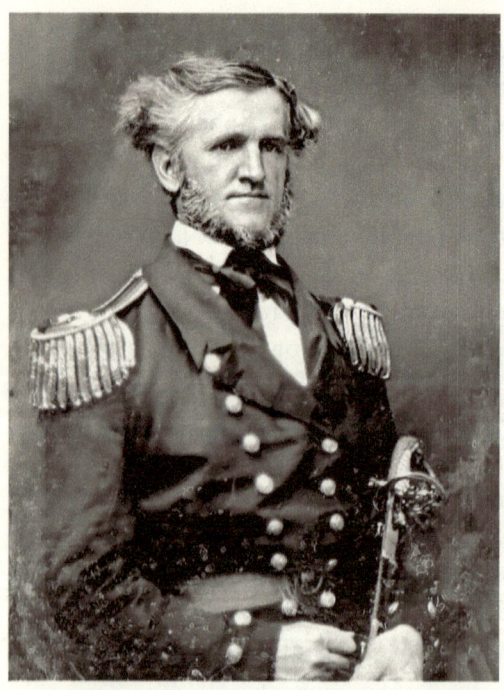

Antebellum image of Lewis W. Minor, who resigned as a USN surgeon in April 1861 and served briefly in Virginia's navy. While in the CSN, Minor served as surgeon of station at Mobile and New Orleans (courtesy Jonathan O'Neal, M.D.).

showed him as "not on duty (sick)," or "unemployed." He appears never to have served in the CSN.[15]

With the exception of the Georgia (in whose navy Thomas J. Charlton, Jr., served) and Virginia, it appears that the only other state whose navy contributed one or more medical officers to the CSN was South Carolina. Robert R. Gibbes reported for duty as a medical officer with that navy on January 6, 1861, examined recruits, and served on the receiving ship *Rattlesnake*, steamer *Excel*, guard boat *Gordon*, and steamer *William Seabrook*. After the South Carolina navy was disbanded, Gibbes served in the CSN, being first posted to CSS *Lady Davis* in late May 1861. Physician James M. Pelot was appointed surgeon in South Carolina's navy, served on CSS *Lady Davis* when it captured the vessel *A.B. Thompson* on May 19, 1861, and was listed as an assistant surgeon receiving a share of the resulting prize money. Although he later served as an assistant surgeon in the Confederate army, he is not known to have been commissioned as a CSN medical officer. Other medical officers from state navies who later served as army surgeons included Wyatt M. Brown and Alexander Y.P. Garnett. In addition, Edward Warren, a prominent civilian physician, was appointed surgeon-in-chief of North Carolina's navy but grew bored with his "uneventful service" and sought "real surgical work" in the Confederate army.[16]

One state-associated organization that lasted until the end of the war was the Texas Marine Department, an element of the Confederate army's District of Texas, New Mexico, and Arizona. The Marine Department, which consisted of vessels used principally to defend the Texas coast and provide logistical support, employed various physicians—J.A. Barnett, William Boyd, and F.W. Stephens, for example—none of whom are known to have been commissioned officers in the Confederate navy or army.[17]

Overall Contribution of the USN

The CSN's resources and activities did grow over time, as did its need for medical officers. In all, 51 medical officers resigned or were dismissed from the USN from December 1, 1860, to December 1, 1863, with 37 being commissioned—that is, appointed by the president, with congressional approval—in the medical corps of the CSN. The remaining 14, including officers of both Northern and Southern origin, did not receive CSN commissions and can largely be accounted for by the baseline USN resignation rate, among medical officers, of about four per year. Among medical officers leaving the USN were Surgeon Thomas B. Steele and Assistant Surgeon Charles Lowndes, Jr., both from Maryland. The sympathies of both were evidently with the South, and their resignation letters were dated within a day of each other in late April 1861; Steele was allowed to resign, whereas Lowndes was dismissed. Rather than join the Confederate military, both returned to civilian life in Maryland, Steele in Cambridge and Lowndes in Baltimore.[18]

Of the 106 men known to have been appointed as medical officers in the CSN—not all of whom accepted their appointment or served throughout the war—slightly more than a third (the aforementioned 37) had served in the USN (Appendix A). Although they may not ever have entered Federal service, Robert R. Gibbes and Charles M. Morfit had passed the examination to become USN assistant surgeon and received CSN appointments. Not only did former USN physicians form the core of the CSN's new medical service, but their departure also created a temporary void in the ranks of USN surgeons, for that loss accounted for about a quarter of USN positions for medical officers.

With the expansion of the CSN and the appearance that defections from the USN had practically stopped, OMS chief Spotswood realized that a roster comprising just former USN medical officers could not provide an adequate level of service. Clearly, additional physicians would have to be recruited from other sources.

– 3 –

Wanted: More Medical Officers

In light of the modest number of CSN vessels and facilities at the end of 1861, the 21 full surgeons so far commissioned seemed adequate in number. The 12 assistant surgeons, however, were not enough, and consequently, an act approved on December 24, 1861, allowed for the appointment of 30 additional assistant surgeons "from the navy or from civil life." In contrast with the existing appointments, the length of which was undefined, the newly approved appointments would terminate at the end of the war, so the new officers came to be known as "assistant surgeons for the war." The act omitted any mention of how candidates for those positions were to be found or evaluated.[1]

The medical corps responded by publicizing the need for new officers and then subjecting candidates to an examination by a board of surgeons, as was the custom in the USN. The process took time; the first assistant surgeons for the war entered CSN service in mid-March 1862. One of the earliest so appointed was Samuel D. Drewry, a farmer and physician from Virginia, who evidently had no great desire to serve in the military. Drewry, predicting that he would soon be conscripted—the first conscription act was signed into law on April 16, 1862—applied to be a CSN assistant surgeon for the war. After his appointment as such was confirmed on March 26, 1862, he served on various assignments. On October 11, 1862, President Davis approved a bill that exempted various persons from conscription, including physicians who had been in practice for the past five years. That description included Drewry, so he resigned from the CSN and afterward "had no connexion with the Army or Navy." It is not possible to determine how many other men had a similar motive in applying to be CSN medical officers.[2]

Several examination sessions for prospective assistant surgeons—presided over by senior surgeons such as James Cornick and Lewis W. Minor—occurred during the war in various cities, including Richmond, New Orleans, and Macon. Examinations were required for Confederate army medical officers wishing to transfer to the CSN. Similar boards assessed the suitability of CSN assistant surgeons for promotion to surgeon. Except for CSN assistant surgeons who were being evaluated for such promotion, medical officers who had served in the USN were evidently exempt from examination.[3]

Examining Prospective Medical Officers

A spring 1862 newspaper announcement about examinations for prospective CSN assistant surgeons for the war provided few details, other than the facts that candidates had to be between 21 and 30 years of age—in contrast, the required age range in the USN was 21 to 25 years—and must present "proper letters of moral character." However, the CSN generally followed USN practices, and examining boards were chaired by surgeons with long prior service in the USN, so USN procedures probably give a fair picture of how CSN examining boards operated. There is no indication that the evaluation process differed between candidates for temporary (for the war) and permanent appointments.[4]

Men interested in joining the USN medical corps applied to the secretary of the navy, stating their age, birthplace, and residence and including "respectable testimonials" of having the needed moral and physical qualifications. A number of applicants—enough to provide the navy with qualified men to fill the assistant surgeon vacancies likely to occur in the coming year—were invited to appear before an examining board. The invitees underwent a physical examination by one or more board members. On passing that, they signed a preprinted certificate of physical capacity: "I declare, on honor, that my

3. Wanted: More Medical Officers

health at this time is good and robust; and, to the best of my knowledge and belief, I am free from constitutional defects, and without any predisposition to epilepsy, phthisis pulmonalis [tuberculosis], gout, or chronic disease of any kind. I have neither circocele [enlargement of veins within the scrotum], stricture of the urethra, hemorrhoids, nor hernia. Each and all of my organs of sense are without imperfection."[5]

One man who sought an appointment as a CSN medical officer was John R. Bracey, a physician serving as a private in the 14th Virginia Infantry Regiment. One of his letters of support, which praised Bracey's character, acknowledged that he "is by no means blessed with a strong & vigorous constitution, but on the contrary, he has so far been unable to bear the hardships of the camp." Indeed, much of Bracey's service in the infantry was marked by illness before he transferred to the 3rd Virginia Cavalry Regiment. Whether a naval board ever examined him for a possible appointment is not known, but it seems unlikely that he would have been found physically fit. Bracey was killed in July 1864 at Louisa Court House, Virginia, probably during the Battle of Trevilian Station.[6]

Whether graduation from a medical school was required for CSN applicants has not been determined. Among men examined for an appointment as assistant surgeon in the USN during 1861–65, 8.6 percent reported that they were not medical-school graduates, but how the lack of a medical diploma affected their candidacy is unknown. As was the case for the Confederate army, the CSN probably preferred medical officers who embraced allopathic (mainstream or "regular") practice rather a sectarian system such as botanical medicine or homeopathy. Among the allopathic medical schools of the time, most were in the North, with only five Southern schools remaining open after the 1860–61 session. The Union capture of New Orleans prompted the closure of two of those schools, located in Louisiana, after the 1861–62 session. For the 1862–65 sessions, the remaining allopathic schools were MCV, with 191 graduates; the University of Nashville, with 75; and the University of Virginia, with five. Many physicians of the time practiced without having a medical diploma. Attending a medical school often required no more than the payment of lecture fees, and graduation typically required attendance of two sessions of lectures, which were usually identical if given at the same school, with each session lasting several months. Many practitioners attended one lecture session only.[7]

Assistant surgeon applicants answered, in writing, a series of medical questions and appeared in person to be interviewed before the board, which before the war typically met annually and consisted of at least three medical officers, usually with one acting as a recorder. In March 1860, Robert R. Gibbes presented himself before an USN examining board in Philadelphia. His preserved examination materials include a signed certificate of physical capacity and handwritten documents including an autobiography, an essay (thesis) on a topic assigned by the board—Gibbes's was on opium—and short answers to a series of written questions. The 12 written questions posed to Gibbes included "Explain the difference between congestion & inflammation," "Write a prescription for pills of calomel, digitalis and squill," and "What are the common properties of matter?"[8]

The USN board examining Gibbes employed a ranking system, perhaps similar to one used in 1854 that had applicants evaluated in 11 fields: (1) physical qualifications, (2) medical school, (3) general aptitude, (4) literary and scientific acquirements, (5) anatomy and physiology, (6) principles and practice of surgery, (7) principles and practice of medicine, (8) obstetrics, (9) materia medica (the therapeutic properties of medicines), (10) chemistry, and (11) medical jurisprudence. In the 1854 scale, the fields of physical qualifications and medical school were the only ones not scored numerically. Maximum scores for the other fields were 40 points each for obstetrics and medical jurisprudence and 100 each for the remaining seven areas, for a maximum possible aggregate score of 780 points. Also taken into consideration were overall merit and the candidate's performance on his assigned thesis. An acceptable candidate had to receive an aggregate score of at least 540 points, with a minimum of 20 points each in obstetrics and medical jurisprudence, 50 points each in materia medica and chemistry, and 80 points each for the remaining five areas. Candidates with the highest scores, provided

3. Wanted: More Medical Officers

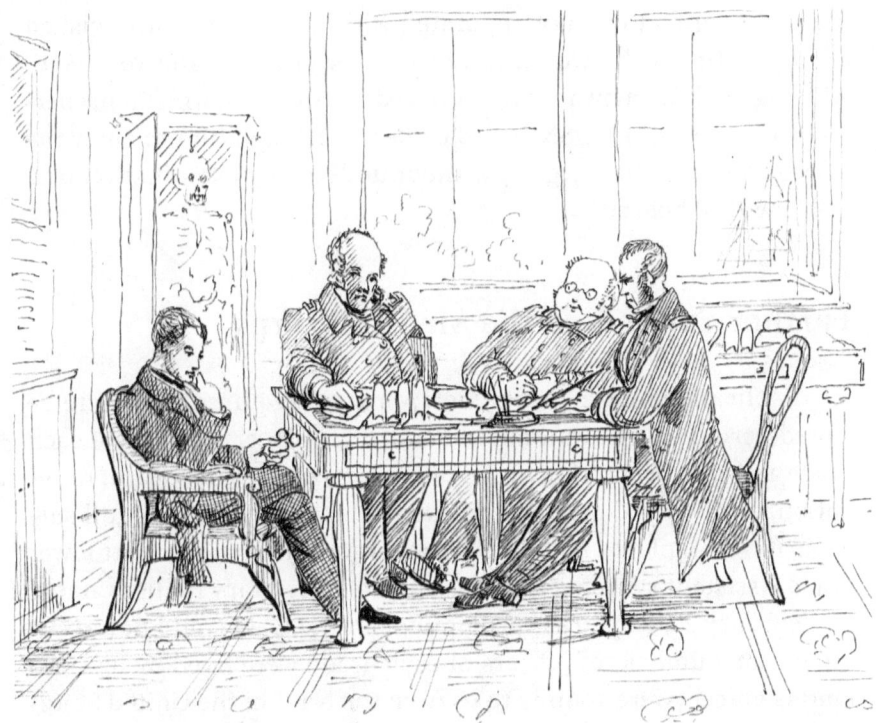

Sketch by Charles Ellery Stedman showing himself (far left) being examined during the Civil War by naval surgeons (caricatured and unidentified) for an appointment as an assistant surgeon in the USN. The examination process in the CSN was probably similar (Civil War Photograph Collection, Vol. 14, Military Order of the Loyal Legion of the United States, Massachusetts Commandery [MOLLUS-MASS], U.S. Army Heritage and Education Center, Carlisle, PA [USAHEC]).

they were at least 540 points, were entitled to the first appointments. Members of boards were instructed to report "favorably upon no case admitting of a reasonable doubt, as the health and the lives of the officers and men of the Navy are objects too important to be intrusted to ignorant or incompetent persons."[9]

Gibbes, a South Carolinian, ranked sixth among the seven applicants receiving a satisfactory score, but there were assistant surgeon vacancies for the first four only. Those four included James E. Lindsay and Osborn S. Iglehart, who became USN assistant surgeons later in 1860 and subsequently joined the CSN. If a candidate deemed qualified was not appointed within a year and still wished an appointment, he would have to be reexamined and reranked. Although Gibbes may not have received a USN appointment, his performance before the USN board evidently allowed him to enter the CSN as an assistant surgeon without undergoing examination by a CSN medical board.[10]

Further Expanding the Medical Corps

Replication of the USN seniority system required that there be a predetermined maximum number of CSN officers allowed at each grade and that promotion occur only when promotion, death, resignation, or dismissal created a vacancy in one grade (that of full surgeon, for example) to be filled by the senior officer at the next lower grade (assistant surgeon, in this example). Secretary Mallory noted on February 27, 1862, that promotions in the CSN could not occur unless the numbers of officers of each grade were fixed by law. "So long as officers were coming to us from the Navy of the United States and places were reserved for them this could not be done," said Mallory, "but ample time has been afforded to all who desired to join us from that source." Since the end of 1861, the addition of Surgeons Charles F. Fahs and Richard W. Jeffery—offset by the January 1862 death of Surgeon George Blacknall—had increased the net number of surgeons from 21 to 22, and the addition of Assistant Surgeons James W. Herty and James E. Lindsay had increased the number of officers at that grade from 12 to 14. Mallory indicated that promotion could occur more frequently if the number of grades was increased.[11]

The Confederate Congress, a bicameral body as of February 18, 1862, responded by passing a new bill, approved by President Davis on April 21, 1862, that reset the number of commissioned CSN officers. For the medical corps, 22 surgeons, 15 passed assistant surgeons, and 30 assistant surgeons were allowed; none of those appointments would necessarily terminate at the end of the war. Thus, the grade of passed assistant surgeon—existing in the USN but

3. Wanted: More Medical Officers

heretofore missing from the CSN—was added, and the new number of permanent slots for assistant surgeons (30) meant that 16 more men could be appointed at that latter grade. (The allowed number of assistant surgeons for the war remained unchanged at 30.) All of the slots for passed assistant surgeon could not be filled immediately because to qualify for that grade, a CSN assistant surgeon had to have served for three years, including time in the USN (and possibly in a state navy), and pass an examination. (The corresponding time requirement in the USN was five years of total service, including two years at sea.) Nevertheless, Thomas J. Charlton, Jr., Frederic Garretson, and John W. Sandford, Jr., were promoted to passed assistant surgeon in September 1862, and at least 10 other assistant surgeons were likewise promoted during the remainder of the war. Although no CSN passed assistant surgeon reached the grade of surgeon, attaining the former grade was a true promotion and brought with it higher pay than that received by assistant surgeons.[12]

Examining Assistant Surgeons for Promotion

Again, the USN procedure for promoting assistant surgeons was probably a model for the CSN. USN assistant surgeons applying for promotion presented to the examining board "testimonials of correct deportment and habits of industry from the Surgeons with whom they have been associated on duty; also, a journal of Practice, or Case-Book, in their own hand-writing." They were also expected to be familiar with the duties of medical officers as stated in a USN instruction book. A physical examination was apparently not necessary. Applicants who were ordered to report for examination but failed, without satisfactory reason, to appear or were deemed, after examination, by the board to be "not qualified" for promotion were to be dropped from the navy's list of officers.[13]

Assistant Surgeons Thomas J. Charlton, Jr., and John W. Sandford, Jr., two of the first three CSN medical officers promoted to passed assistant surgeon, were ordered in late May 1862 to proceed from Savannah, where they were stationed, to Macon. There they were to report to Surgeon James Cornick, president of the examining board, and be assessed for their suitability for promotion. They evidently performed satisfactorily, as evidenced by their September 1862 promotion. The third officer promoted at the same time to passed assistant surgeon was Frederic Garretson, but where and by whom he was examined are not known.[14]

Assistant Surgeon Robert R. Gibbes, CSN, was ordered to report to Richmond to be examined, starting on January 15, 1864, for promotion to passed assistant surgeon. Gibbes had first reported for duty in the South Carolina navy on January 9, 1861, and for CSN duty on May 27, 1861, so perhaps his time in the state navy (and any short time in the USN) counted as part of the required three years of service. The examination was postponed until June 1864 and then rescheduled for May. The ordeal, which took place at the Richmond Naval Hospital, was spread over three days, with the examining board consisting of Surgeons James Cornick (president of the board), William B. Sinclair, and James F. Harrison, all of whom had been full surgeons in the USN. On the first day (May 3), Gibbes was told to write a thesis on remittent fever, a task he spent three hours to complete. On the second day, he underwent five hours of oral questioning, with queries from Cornick on anatomy and surgery, Sinclair on physiology and the practice of medicine, and Harrison on chemistry and materia medica. On the final day, Gibbes wrote answers to written questions. A few days later, Gibbes was informed in person that his performance had been satisfactory and that he would be promoted to passed assistant surgeon as soon as the board adjourned. It appears that the same board examined Assistant Surgeon Charles M. Morfit in Richmond in late June 1864.[15]

Working with the New Limits

By the spring of 1862, no additional former USN officers were expected to join the CSN, so the 16 new openings for permanent assistant surgeon allowed by the act of April 21, 1862, would have to be filled from civil life or from the list of assistant surgeons for

3. Wanted: More Medical Officers

the war. On August 26, 1862, before any assistant surgeons had been promoted to passed assistant surgeon, Assistant Surgeon Algernon S. Garnett became the only CSN medical officer promoted to surgeon. The allowed number of full surgeons was capped at 22, but the death of Surgeon Randolph F. Mason in early August 1862 created a vacancy for Garnett, the assistant surgeon with the most seniority.[16]

Although 30 assistant surgeons for the war were permitted at any one time, 52 men were appointed to that grade by the middle of 1864. Of those officers, 24 were converted to assistant surgeons with appointments not limited by the length of the war—a process requiring Senate approval but no additional examination—to help fill the additional openings created by the act of April 21, 1862, and to replace assistant surgeons who had resigned or been promoted to passed assistant surgeon.[17]

On November 30, 1863, Spotswood reported to Secretary Mallory that despite the official limit of 22 surgeons, he now had 23 because William D. Harrison, after a prolonged cruise aboard a USN vessel, had recently left the Union navy to become a Confederate naval surgeon. (Whether exceeding the lawful limit raised any objections is not known.) Because the activities of the navy were increasing, Spotswood recommended expanding the number of surgeons to 30 by promoting some passed assistant surgeons. Full surgeons, said Spotswood, were needed at naval hospitals, where "experienced practical surgeons" were called for, and they should also be assigned to "shore stations and the large vessels [cruisers] that may be brought into commission abroad." Spotswood did not recommend increasing the number of permanent slots for assistant surgeon but did advise increasing the number of assistant surgeons for the war from 30 to 40 to account for "even a moderate increase" of the "Naval Establishment."[18]

Spotswood's call for additional experienced practical surgeons at naval hospitals must be considered in light of the actual clinical expertise that those prospective new surgeons would have had. In late November 1863, the CSN's seven most seasoned passed assistant surgeons—the number needed to bring the number of full surgeons to 30—had entered the USN as assistant surgeons between May 1857 and August 1859. Although four to six years of experience was substantial, it was much less than what Spotswood had been accustomed to in the USN. Just before the war started, for example, the seven USN passed assistant surgeons first in line for promotion—after excluding those later judged unfit—had entered the USN as assistant surgeons in 1847 and thus had a least a decade more experience that the CSN's most senior passed assistant surgeons. Yet the CSN's passed assistant surgeons had been deemed qualified for promotion, and the war forced Spotswood to work with the personnel he had.[19]

On April 28, 1864, Spotswood repeated his call to Secretary Mallory for more surgeons, because important posts requiring such officers now existed—for example, the fortifications at Drewry's Bluff, Virginia; the hospital at Smithville, North Carolina; and the ironclad steamer *Virginia II*. If the navy intended that a full surgeon be assigned to each ironclad vessel, said Spotswood, then the number should be increased to at least 30.[20]

Although Spotswood's requests were fruitless, he did receive modest assistance as a result of the Confederate Congress creating the Provisional Navy of the Confederate States (PNCS) on May 1, 1863. That action was largely an attempt to allow the promotion of young energetic line officers and to circumvent some of the restrictions imposed by the traditional seniority system. Men could be appointed to the PNCS from the regular navy at their current grade and seniority while keeping their position in the regular navy, but PNCS commissions would expire when the war ended; the PNCS would also accept appointees from civil life. Because there was no limit on the number of PNCS officers at each grade, officers who proved their worthiness for a higher grade would not have to wait for a vacancy to be promoted. If an officer held appointments in both the regular navy and the PNCS and was promoted in the latter only, he would retain his lower regular-navy grade when the war ended and the PNCS was disbanded.[21]

For more than a year, the act creating the PNCS spurred almost no action. Then in June 1864, most officers in the regular navy were appointed to the PNCS, an action that had little effect on the manpower of the medical corps. However, during fall 1864, PNCS

3. Wanted: More Medical Officers

appointments as assistant surgeon were granted to eight new men, who—because the PNCS would disband when the war ended—were effectively assistant surgeons for the war. Shortly before their appointment, the corps had men filling 28 of the 30 slots for assistant surgeon for the war. Thus, the new PNCS appointments brought the medical corps roster of assistant surgeons for the war up to 36, six more than its previously allowed limit.[22]

On November 1, 1864, in his final published report to Mallory, Surgeon Spotswood again asked that the number of surgeons be increased, to at least 28 or 30. Full surgeons, said Spotswood, were needed at several places, especially the Mobile Squadron, where only one surgeon was on duty because the other surgeon assigned to the station was absent on sick leave. Spotswood also wanted a full surgeon to assist him in the OMS, which was mostly "under the charge of newly appointed assistant surgeons." Spotswood indicated that he had fewer than the allowed number of passed assistant surgeons because most assistant surgeons had not served long enough to qualify for the surgeons' examination. He deemed the number of assistant surgeons with permanent appointments and with appointments for the war sufficient for the time being. Spotswood's request again produced no useful response.[23]

Spotswood's long-standing requests to increase the allowed number of full surgeons imply that he hoped that legislation would make those additional slots available. However, the same goal—having enough qualified officers to fill assignments suitable for full surgeons—could have been attained in at least two other ways. First, some or all of the passed assistant surgeons in the regular navy could have been promoted to surgeon in the PNCS. That action, which was possible immediately after the PNCS was created in May 1863, would have required only that President Davis recommend the promotions and the Senate confirm them. Second, changes could have been made to the rules that governed the types of assignments that the various grades of medical officers could fill. Those rules, documentation of which has not been found, were created by the Navy Department, as shown by Spotswood's remark that requiring a full surgeon on all ironclad vessels was for the department to decide. Since examining boards had deemed passed assistant surgeons to be qualified for duty as full surgeons, it could be argued that distinctions between the two grades—with respect to their assignments—were artificial and should be removed. Spotswood, then, could have tried to convince Secretary Mallory to recommend the promotion of passed assistant surgeons to full surgeons in the PNCS or to allow passed assistant surgeons to assume responsibilities previously reserved for full surgeons. Whether Spotswood pursued either course has not been determined.[24]

Contribution of the Confederate Army

Spotswood was probably surprised that the major source of medical officers for the CSN was not the USN but rather the Confederate army, which accounted for no fewer than 47 appointees. The plurality had been army assistant surgeons or surgeons, although at least 10 had been privates; it was not unusual for physicians to serve in the ranks instead of as medical officers. Others had been acting assistant surgeons (civilian contract surgeons) or held the position of hospital steward, a grade of noncommissioned officer with apothecary and other medical duties. The opposite—moving from the CSN to the Confederate army—also occurred. At least six men appointed as a medical officer in the CSN were afterward appointed in the Confederate army as a surgeon, assistant surgeon, or contract surgeon. The acceptance of an army appointment would have required those men to decline or resign their CSN appointment, but such documentation, although presumed to have been created, has not been found for Walter E. Bondurant and John C. Harrison. Bondurant was an artillery private before serving as a CSN assistant surgeon for the war, after which he was appointed assistant surgeon in the army. Similarly, Harrison served as an infantry private and worked as an army contract surgeon before being appointed assistant surgeon for the war in the CSN; he was later an assistant surgeon in the army. The net gain for the CSN medical corps from men changing military branches was about 40.[25]

3. Wanted: More Medical Officers

Resignation letters generally indicated little about physicians' reasons for leaving the army for an appointment in the CSN. Some probably sought a different type of military service in another setting, and those with health problems may have believed that a naval assignment might make recovery more likely. Surgeon James Grey Thomas of the 19th Regiment of North Carolina Troops (2nd Cavalry) tendered his resignation on October 27, 1862, stating that the climate—he was stationed at Warrenton, Virginia—made him physically unable to perform his duties; he wished to go to Havana, Cuba, immediately. A committee of army surgeons reported that Thomas had a serious case of bronchitis and should not remain in camp through the upcoming winter. Assistant Surgeon Hugh S. Paisley of the 19th Alabama Infantry Regiment tendered his resignation on May 20, 1863, citing prolonged illness. An examining surgeon verified that Paisley suffered from chronic diarrhea and hemorrhoids and that generally poor health made him unfit for duty. Thomas and Paisley entered the CSN as assistant surgeons for the war in April 1864. Details of Thomas's service and health while in the CSN are not available, and limited information about Paisley shows him on shore duty in South Carolina.[26]

The Confederate army required that medical officers who had entered the service without having passed a qualifying examination be subject to such an examination to ensure their fitness to serve. It is possible that failing that examination, or unwillingness to take it, drove some army medical officers to seek a CSN appointment even if that route required a passing grade from a naval examining board. Others may have preferred the navy, applied at about the same time to both branches, and accepted an army appointment before learning that the navy was also offering a position. In at least one case, a disciplinary action may have driven the move from army to navy. After Surgeon General Moore of the army learned that Assistant Surgeon William W. Coggin had accepted money for examining substitutes for conscripted men, Coggin was dropped from the rolls of the army on December 21, 1863. Coggin appealed the decision and asked that his punishment might at least be made less severe, but he was unsuccessful, and the best he could do was to obtain as position as an army contract surgeon, in which capacity he was serving by September 1864. Coggin then applied for an appointment as assistant surgeon in the CSN, and his nomination and Senate confirmation for that position occurred on November 10 and 23, 1864, respectively.[27]

Former army hospital stewards Luther R. Dickinson and William D. Sale graduated in 1864 from MCV in Richmond. They may have taken advantage of a practice, described by Surgeon General Moore, by which the army medical department assigned selected hospital stewards and other men with apparent medical aptitude to duty in Richmond and allowed them attend lectures at the college. Upon graduation (sometimes before), such individuals were invited to appear before an examining board for appointment as medical officers. Private Cincinnatus M. Parker, from a Mississippi infantry regiment, was detached to perform medical duties in Richmond, apparently without ever being appointed as a hospital steward. There he attended MCV, graduated in 1863, and entered the CSN as an assistant surgeon in May 1863.[28]

Although Moore undoubtedly expected the men he allowed to attend MCV to apply for the army medical corps, it is unclear whether seeking a CSN appointment was discouraged. In fact, resignations from the army seemed to be readily accepted when the reason given was to accept a CSN appointment. Assistant Surgeon William Mason Turner of the army sought a CSN appointment and learned from Secretary Mallory that although resignation from the army was not needed for him to take the CSN examination, it was a prerequisite for receiving CSN orders. Mallory also told Turner that he would need written permission from the secretary of war, which was granted, to appear before the CSN examining board.[29]

Manpower Peak of the CSN Medical Corps

As far as can be determined—CSN records after 1864 are scarce—the naval medical corps was at its peak strength around December 1, 1864, with 90 officers: 22 surgeons, 12 passed assistant surgeons (in the regular navy or PNCS), 27 assistant surgeons with

3. Wanted: More Medical Officers

permanent appointments, and 29 assistant surgeons whose appointments were for the duration of the war (Appendix A). In all, 106 men are known to have been appointed as CSN medical officers. Among the 16 not serving on December 1, 1864, six had died (George Blacknall, Daniel S. Green, Randolph F. Mason, Joseph D. Grafton, Jr., David E. Ewart, and William T. Williams), six had left the CSN for Confederate army service (Robert T. Baldwin, Jr., Walter E. Bondurant, Samuel L. Bonner, John C. Harrison, Henry Stone, and John Ward), and two had resigned their CSN appointment without entering army service (John Joseph Steinriede and Samuel D. Drewry). The remaining two, Hodijah B. Meade and Henry Christmas, served as assistant surgeons in the CSA before being appointed to the CSN as assistant surgeons for the war—Christmas had even been promoted to assistant surgeon, CSN—but declined their CSN appointments and continued in the CSA. Not all of the 90 medical officers on the rolls on December 1, 1864, were available for duty. At least three—Passed Assistant Surgeon Thomas J. Charlton, Jr., and Assistant Surgeons Thomas Emory and Joseph S. Tipton—were being held as prisoners of war, and others may have been too ill to serve. The number of civilian physicians employed by the CSN has not been determined.[30]

In comparison, the USN had on January 1, 1865, 188 active medical officers in the regular navy and 228 temporary medical officers called acting assistant surgeons. The latter, members of the USN's so-called volunteer—as opposed to regular—service, were the counterparts of the CSN's assistant surgeons for the war or assistant surgeons in the PNCS. (In contrast, in the U.S. Army and Confederate army and navy, "acting assistant surgeon" usually referred to a civilian physician on temporary duty, often called a contract surgeon.) The CSN's medical corps was also dwarfed when compared with that of the Confederate army, which appears to have had more than 3,000 surgeon and assistant surgeon positions that were filled throughout the war, because of turnover, by as many as 7,400 men, not including contract surgeons.[31]

* * *

The Confederate Navy Medical Corps

The modest size of the CSN's medical corps reflected the South's resources, the limitations that were consequently placed on Confederate naval strategy, and the fact that the nature of the war mandated that army would consume a much greater portion of the South's manpower and materiel. There was, in fact, both competition and cooperation between the medical services of the Confederate army and navy for officers and supplies, and the higher priority given the army contributed to repeated efforts by naval officers to elevate their status to equal that of their army brethren. Understanding that quest for parity requires an understanding of the place of naval officers in the military establishment.

– 4 –

Standing of Naval Medical Officers

Where naval medical officers stood among other commissioned naval officers, and in relation to their army brethren, was a long-standing concern in the USN that carried over into the CSN. Commissioned officers—those appointed by the president with congressional approval—were divided into line and staff officers. Line officers were eligible for command afloat and could be thought of as those whose primary duty was to engage the enemy. In the CSN, the commissioned officer grades at the war's onset were, in descending order, captain, commander, and lieutenant. Officers' order of precedence, or rank, within each grade, was determined by the date they assumed their current grade and, after that, the date they assumed lower grades. In April 1862, admirals, ranking above captains, were added; lieutenants were divided into first and second lieutenants; and masters in line of promotion, ranking below second lieutenants, were added as commissioned officers. Also belonging to the line were certain warrant officers—appointed by the secretary of the navy—including masters (other than those in line of promotion) and midshipmen. Staff officers, including surgeons, paymasters, engineers, and others, were commissioned but auxiliary to the line and could not hold naval command. Staff officers had a grade, such as surgeon or assistant surgeon, but that classification did not indicate their place relative to line officers.[1]

Assimilated and Relative Rank

The relative standing of CSN medical officers with respect to CSN line officers—which was important for purposes of protocol and social status in the tradition-bound navy—was put forth in documents that assigned *assimilated rank* to staff officers. An April 1864 summary provided by Commander John K. Mitchell, chief of the Office of Orders and Detail, indicted that the assimilated rank of a surgeon with more than 12 years of service (including USN service) was commander, that of a surgeon with less service was first lieutenant, that of a passed assistant surgeon was between second lieutenant and master, and that of an assistant surgeon was passed midshipman.[2]

CSN specifications for uniforms—probably issued before April 1862, when the grade of admiral was added and lieutenants were split into first and second lieutenants—were generally consistent with Mitchell's summary. From a distance, the strips of gold lace on the coat cuffs were probably the most obvious indicator of rank or grade. Although the topmost strip for a flag officer (not a formal grade), captain, commander, and lieutenant had a loop—that for medical officers did not—the number and width of strips were the same for commanders and surgeons with at least 12 years of service (two strips, each a half-inch wide), for lieutenants and surgeons with less than 12 years of service (one strip, a half-inch wide), and for masters and passed assistant surgeons (one strip, a quarter-inch wide). Passed midshipmen and assistant surgeons both had three medium-sized naval buttons, but no lace strips, on the cuff. The design of shoulder straps differed substantially between line and medical officers and implied little about assimilated rank. Captains and surgeons with at least 12 years of service had three stars on their cap device, commanders and surgeons with less service had two, lieutenants and passed assistant surgeons had one, and masters and assistant surgeons had none. Whatever the regulation uniforms suggested about assimilated rank, officers who had been in the USN often preferred wearing their old blue uniforms—perhaps now displaying their respective state or CSN buttons—in part because it was expensive to outfit oneself in a new regulation steel-gray CSN uniform. Indicators of CSN grade appearing in period photographs sometimes differ from those put forth in the official uniform specifications.[3]

How Confederate army and naval grades related to each other,

4. Standing of Naval Medical Officers

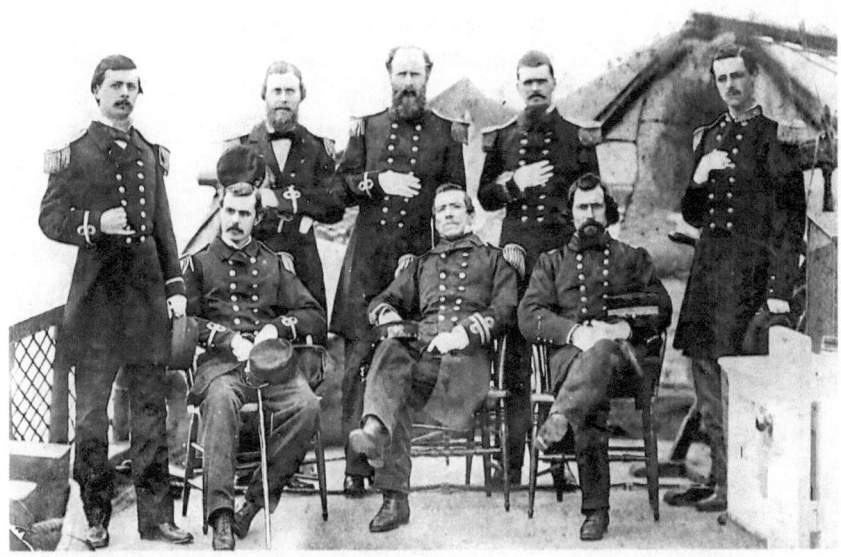

Confederate officers on the deck of CSS *Sumter* in 1861 or 1862. Standing, from left, are Surgeon Francis L. Galt; Lieutenants John M. Stribling, John M. Kell, and Robert T. Chapman; and First Lieutenant Becket K. Howell (Marine Corps). Seated, from left, are Lieutenant William E. Evans, Commander Raphael Semmes, and First Assistant Engineer Miles J. Freeman. According to uniform regulations, the lace strips on the sleeves of the naval line officers should not have a lower loop, and the strips on Galt's sleeves should have no loops at all (Naval History and Heritage Command, Washington, D.C. [NHHC], image NH 42383).

relative rank, had been left for the president to determine. It was widely considered through most of the war—although evidently not put forth officially—that a naval commander ranked with an army major, a naval lieutenant with an army captain, and a naval master with an army first lieutenant. The first official decree on relative rank was an act of February 16, 1864, which specified the army and naval grades that would receive the same allowances for rations, quarters, and fuel. Allowances could be identical for grades adjacent to each other, so the act provided rough guidance rather than grade-for-grade equivalents. According to Commander Mitchell's summary, allowances for naval surgeons (with any length of service) equaled those for army lieutenant colonels and majors, and those for naval passed assistant surgeons and assistant surgeons equaled those for army first and second lieutenants. In February 1865, President Davis issued an order establishing relative ranks between officers in the PNCS and those in the Provisional Army of the Confederate States (PACS), the for-the-war counterpart of the PNCS. That order, when combined with the April 1864 summary of assimilated rank, made PNCS surgeons with more than 12 years of service equivalent to PACS majors, and PNCS surgeons with less service equivalent to PACS captains. PNCS passed assistant surgeons ranked between PACS first and second lieutenants, and PNCS assistant surgeons ranked with PACS cadets.[4]

One additional consideration was how Confederate naval and army medical officers compared with respect to the relationship between grade and length of service. In the regular (permanent) army, a surgeon, regardless of length of service, had an actual grade of major, and an assistant surgeon had an actual grade of captain. In the PACS, which was to be disbanded at the war's termination and contained the vast majority of army officers, surgeons and assistant surgeons had the assimilated rank of major and captain, respectively. Regardless of how one interpreted the confusing official declarations touching on assimilated and relative rank, it was clear that a naval assistant surgeon was at least a grade lower than an army assistant surgeon. Another prominent difference was that Surgeon Spotswood, chief of the navy's OMS, had an assimilated rank of commander and relative rank of army lieutenant colonel and occupied those levels only because of his long naval service. Spotswood's position could actually have been assigned to an assistant surgeon at a much lower relative rank. In contrast, Spotswood's counterpart in the army's medical department was the surgeon general, who had an actual rank of colonel.[5]

Naval medical officers could also compare their salaries with those in the army. Although pay depended on length and type of service, a new CSN assistant surgeon, at the beginning of the war, received $1,050 a year if not on sea duty, whereas a new army assistant surgeon received $1,320. A newly appointed CSN surgeon not on sea duty received $2,000 a year, which was comparable to the $1,944

4. Standing of Naval Medical Officers

salary of a new army surgeon. However, appointment as a naval surgeon required at least three years of service as an assistant surgeon—the actual time was usually much longer—whereas many full surgeons in the PACS were appointed directly from civilian life.[6]

Fleet Surgeons

The pay of CSN medical officers increased with their length of naval service and when they served at sea, but otherwise, their actual duty assignment typically had no effect on salary. The one exception appears to have been assignment as a fleet surgeon, who was a medical officer assigned to the staff of a line officer commanding a squadron (a flag officer). The title of fleet surgeon existed in the USN and was included in CSN regulations and instructions for medical officers, despite it not being a formal grade.[7]

Early in the war, CSN land-based stations and the squadrons associated with them tended to be commanded by the same line officer, who was entitled to have a medical officer on his staff. Although that line officer was simultaneously a station commandant and flag officer, his medical staff officer received neither additional pay nor a formal title, although he was sometimes termed "surgeon of station" or something similar. The first Confederate medical officer given the title of fleet surgeon appears to have been Surgeon Daniel S. Green, who was appointed temporary fleet surgeon of the James River Squadron on December 13, 1862.[8]

On learning of that appointment, Admiral Franklin Buchanan, station commandant and flag officer at Mobile, asked on December 29 that Surgeon Lewis W. Minor, surgeon of station at Mobile, also be appointed fleet surgeon:

> Surgeon Minor has been performing the duties of "Fleet Surgeon" since he has been attached to this station; and as Surgeon Green has received that appointment [for the James River Squadron], I respectfully ask that the appointment be also conferred upon Dr. Minor. The surgeons of our Navy generally are officers of high professional attainments, have served their country faithfully and deserve advancement with other grades. The position of Fleet Surgeon is an important one, and one to which all aspire.

The Confederate Navy Medical Corps

> Although we have no Fleets, and but small Squadron[s] at present in the Confederacy, the medical department of the various vessels require the same supervision of a "Fleet Surgeon" as if they were larger.[9]

Minor had indeed taken on the duties of a fleet surgeon. On December 23, 1862, for example, he approved expenses for medicines needed for CSS *Morgan* of the Mobile Squadron. Nevertheless, Buchanan's request was not approved, and Minor continued to receive his pay of $2,800 per year, which reflected his being a full surgeon for more than 20 years.[10]

However, it appears that medical officers thereafter assigned to perform the duties of a fleet surgeon—including those also serving as surgeons of station—were indeed designated as fleet surgeons. In February 1864, for example, Secretary Mallory, through the Office of Orders and Details, ordered Surgeon James W.B. Greenhow to report to Captain William F. Lynch, flag officer of the North Carolina Squadron, "for duty as 'Fleet Surgeon' of the Naval forces under his command in addition to your duties as Surgeon of the Station." It has not been determined whether the offices of surgeon of station and fleet surgeon were ever filled by separate men at the same locale, but granting the title of fleet surgeon to men who served in both capacities seems only just. If that did not happen, then a medical officer who performed the duties of both a surgeon of station and fleet surgeon but did not have the latter title, as was the case for Minor, would receive less pay than a fleet surgeon who had no station responsibilities.[11]

Assignment as a fleet surgeon could increase one's pay substantially. Daniel B. Conrad, for example, had entered the USN in 1854 and was promoted to passed assistant surgeon in 1860. After leaving the USN in May 1861, he was appointed surgeon in the CSN and received a salary of $2,000 yearly while not on sea duty, the lowest amount possible for a full surgeon. Once Conrad was appointed fleet surgeon for the Mobile Squadron in April 1864, he was entitled to $3,300 yearly for as long as he held that position. In comparison, OMS chief Spotswood—who had about 26 more years of naval service and 21 more years as a full surgeon than Conrad—received $2,800 per year.[12]

4. Standing of Naval Medical Officers

This quirk in pay was primarily the result of the CSN copying most of the USN pay scale but not replicating the USN practice of paying its chief of medicine and surgery an annual salary of $3,500, the highest amount possible for a medical officer. Instead, Spotswood earned the standard salary for a surgeon with at least 20 years at his current grade who was neither serving at sea nor appointed as a fleet surgeon; he received no additional remuneration for this role as the OMS chief. In addition, some of the men who were appointed CSN fleet surgeons, including Conrad, had left the USN as passed assistant surgeons and entered the CSN before it created that grade. They were thus appointed full surgeons in the CSN, which represented a swifter promotion and pay raise than they would have gotten had they remained in the USN during peacetime. Finally, fleet surgeons served much of their time afloat, and sea duty warranted additional pay whatever the grade of officer. The oldest surgeons in the CSN, of whom Spotswood was one, were usually assigned to shore duty and received only their base salary. Whether Spotswood resented being paid less than some of his subordinates has not been determined, but unhappiness over perceived injustices regarding seniority was common among long-serving naval officers. The fact that Spotswood received no additional pay for his highly responsible role may reflect the initial modest expectations that Confederate legislators had for whichever officer would serve as the OMS chief.[13]

Some medical officers believed that the CSN should add fleet surgeon as a formal grade for officers at high levels of command. That concept appeared in various pieces of proposed legislation.

Legislation on Standing of Medical Officers

Numerous bills dealing with the standing of naval officers were introduced in the Confederate Congress only to be put aside without enactment. A Senate bill "for the reorganization of the Navy" (S. 93), introduced on September 22, 1862, called for 20 surgeons, 30 "first assistant surgeons," and 30 "second assistant surgeons," with the sum, 80, being smaller than the current allowance of 97 (22 surgeons, 15 passed assistant surgeons, 30 assistant surgeons, and 30 assistant surgeons for the war). (In the bill, "first assistant surgeons" probably meant "passed assistant surgeons," while "second assistant surgeons" applied to assistant surgeons who had not passed the surgeons' examination.) The bill made a special point of specifying the army grades with which naval grades would correspond, but it did not address how the grades of naval staff officers would correspond with those of naval line officers. The bill was referred to the Senate's Committee on Naval Affairs but progressed no further.[14]

A Senate bill "for the reorganization of the Medical Corps of the Confederate States Navy" (S. 20), introduced on January 28, 1863, deserves special attention because it was supported by and dealt specifically with medical officers. The bill's intent was addressed in an undated broadside published by an unnamed group of medical officers and an undated text of the bill. The handbill bemoaned the lower standing of CSN medical officers compared with their army counterparts. It also proposed grades of naval medical officers along with their assimilated (naval) rank: (1) medical purveyor and fleet surgeons, ranking as captains, (2) surgeons, ranking as commanders, and (3) assistant surgeons, ranking as lieutenants, without indicating whether first or second lieutenant was meant. Except for the medical purveyor, expressed in the singular and presumably intending one officer at that grade, the number of officers at the other grades was not mentioned. The broadside also called for the commanding officer—except for a warrant or petty officer not in the line of promotion—of any vessel, port, or station to have precedence, regardless of grade, over all medical officers attached to the command. Medical officers would share in prize money and have all other honors of their assimilated rank. They would also be part of the court when a medical officer was tried by court-martial.[15]

The broadside made no specific mention of the chief of the OMS, unless that office was equivalent to medical purveyor. The authors may have been recalling that the OMS chief's specific official responsibility was to "make all purchases of medicines and medical supplies for the navy," which was the charge of a medical purveyor. (The OMS chief was also to "perform such other duties appertaining to

4. Standing of Naval Medical Officers

the medical department as the secretary may from time to time direct," but that charge could apply to any naval officer.) In that document, fleet surgeon was recognized as a formal grade above that of surgeon.[16]

The bill's text, which refined and expanded on the handbill's wording, called for four grades of medical officer: (1) a director general (the chief of the OMS) with a relative rank of army brigadier general, (2) 10 inspectors of hospitals and fleets—one to supervise all naval hospitals and the others to act as fleet surgeons—appointed from the grade of surgeon and holding the relative rank of army colonel, (3) 20 surgeons with the relative rank of army major, and (4) 40 assistant surgeons with the relative rank of army captain. In omitting mention of assistant surgeons for the war, the bill effectively reduced the number of allowed medical officers from 97 to 71.[17]

The bill—evidently drawing on a recently introduced USN practice—also allowed elderly or infirm medical officers to be placed on a retired list with reduced pay, with their vacancies to be filled by promotion. (The USN's retired list was allowed by legislation enacted in February, August, and December 1861. By September 1, 1862, multiple surgeons and passed assistant surgeons had been placed on the list.) Assistant surgeons would be eligible for promotion after three years of service, at least two of which had to be on a war vessel in active service; part of the remaining year was to be spent serving in a naval hospital. The broadside's provisions dealing with the precedence of commanding officers, the honors of assimilated rank, and participation in courts-martial were repeated in the bill. An additional provision—added with the approval of Secretary Mallory "for the purpose of removing a difficulty which existed in reference to the pay of medical officers who refused commissions in the Lincoln Navy"—called for service performed in the USN by medical officers currently in the CSN to be counted when computing service length. (Pay at the various grades of CSN medical officer depended on the date of commission, but it had apparently been unclear whether that included USN commissions.)[18]

Among sections of the broadside and bill that were directly comparable, the bill differed in elevating the OMS chief (the director general) above all other medical officers, in creating a director of hospitals (one of the inspectors), and in specifying the total number of medical officers, which was smaller than that already allowed. The bill was presented to and endorsed by numerous high-ranking line officers and given to Secretary Mallory, who expressed no opinion other than adding the provision about the inclusion of previous USN service. After being referred to the Senate's Committee on Naval Affairs, the bill was tabled.[19]

In late January 1863, a Senate bill (S. 15) "for the reorganization of the Navy of the Confederate States, to establish and equalize the grade of officers, and for other purposes" was introduced. The bill, whose wording has not been found, was immediately referred to the Senate Committee on Naval Affairs and tabled in March 1863.[20]

A House bill, possibly identical or similar to S. 15, was introduced in February 1863 (H.R. 15, "An act for the establishment and equalization of the grade of officers of the Navy of the Confederate States, and for other purposes"). Its major implication for medical officers was the establishment of corresponding grades between the navy and army. The House and Senate could not agree on final wording, and H.R. 15 was eventually tabled at the end of April 1863.[21]

Finally, bills with similar titles were introduced in the Senate in January 1864 (S. 189, "A bill for the establishment and equalization of the grades of officers of the Navy, and for other purposes"), the House in February 1864 (undetermined bill number, "A bill for the establishment and equalization of grades of officers of the Navy of the Confederate States"), the Senate in May 1864 (S. 2, "A bill for the establishment and equalization of the grades of officers of the Navy, and for other purposes"), and the House in May 1864 (H.R. 104, a bill "for the establishment and equalization of the grades of officers of the Navy, and for other purposes"). Although the text of the House bills has not been found, that of the Senate bills survives. All four of these bills were referred to the respective Committees on Navy Affairs and failed to progress further.[22]

Senate bill S. 189, introduced on January 16, 1864, near the end of the fourth and final session of the first permanent congress, was revived in slightly modified form as S. 2, which was introduced on

4. Standing of Naval Medical Officers

May 4, 1864, shortly after commencement of the first session of the second congress. Bill S. 2 had a few provisions relevant to medical officers. First, promotion was to be based on seniority, and officers considered for promotion were subject to examination by a board for their fitness. Officers found unfit for promotion because of age, wounds, or infirmity were to be retired and receive leave-of-absence pay, while those found unfit because of inefficiency or incompetency were to be retired on furlough pay, which was lower than leave-of-absence pay. Second, medical officers were to consist of one surgeon in chief, four surgeons of stations or fleet surgeons (one of whom was to be the medical purveyor), 20 surgeons, 12 passed assistant surgeons, and 25 assistant surgeons. Because assistant surgeons for the war were omitted, the bill would have reduced the allowed number of medical officers from 97 to 62. Third, the chief surgeon, surgeons, and assistant surgeons would rank with "officers of similar rank in the army"—that is, with the army's surgeon general, surgeons, and assistant surgeons, respectively—but the bill did not comment on the relative rank of fleet surgeons or the pay of any of the proposed grades. The existing pay scale included all of the proposed grades of medical officer except for the surgeon in chief, so S. 2 did nothing to correct the anomaly of fleet surgeons being paid more than the surgeon in chief.[23]

Another peculiarity of S. 2 was that it made "fleet surgeon" synonymous with "surgeon of station" and considered it a grade instead of a title for the supervisory medical officer of a station or squadron. The bill provided that one of the four fleet surgeons would be the medical purveyor but did not describe the responsibilities of the other three. By mid–1864, the CSN had four fleet surgeons—serving with the James River, North Carolina, Charleston, and Mobile Squadrons—and an undetermined number of surgeons of station, so had the bill been enacted with no changes in assignment, all but three of those officers would have lost their titles, and at least one fleet surgeon would have lost the additional pay he had been receiving as such. Enactment of S. 2, without further legislation to address its deficiencies, would have reduced the size of the medical corps considerably while probably creating confusion and dissatisfaction in its ranks.

The Provisional Navy

Although the 1863 act creating the PNCS did not so state, naval policy required an officer be in the PNCS to serve afloat. PNCS appointments were thus withheld from senior line officers who were thought to be inefficient but would, in the absence of the PNCS, still have been entitled to prestigious commands at sea. Furthermore, President Davis believed that a man could not be assigned to the PNCS unless he was currently serving afloat. For a shore-based officer who wished to serve afloat, that interpretation presented a no-win situation, for he needed a PNCS appointment to do so, but his shore assignment made getting a PNCS appointment impossible. (Davis's dictum was not strictly enforced.) One apparent aim of allowing officers to retain their regular-navy rank was to spare their feelings should they not receive a PNCS appointment. They would, after all, still be in the permanent navy after the war ended, when the PNCS would no longer exist. However, many officers omitted from the PNCS believed they had been snubbed and shelved. Furthermore, the fact that some line officers were not so appointed was problematic in that assignments for sea duty could not be filled quickly from PNCS officers alone.[24]

For the medical corps, the formation of the PNCS had little practical effect. Of the medical officers known to be on duty in June 1864, only 12—all full surgeons, primarily those with the most seniority who had spent most or all of war on shore duty—were omitted from the PNCS. Assistant surgeons for the war entered the PNCS as assistant surgeons, but their naval service would still end at the war's termination. All other medical officers entering the PNCS in June 1864 did so at the same grade they held in the regular navy. Two assistant surgeons in the PNCS and regular navy, Robert R. Gibbes and Charles M. Morfit, were promoted in November 1864 to passed assistant surgeon in the PNCS. There is no congressional record of their receiving parallel promotions in the regular navy, but other evidence points to both officers having been so promoted. Assignments as fleet surgeon, which were prestigious and merited a higher salary, went to PNCS surgeons because non–PNCS surgeons were

4. Standing of Naval Medical Officers

ineligible to serve afloat, but Secretary Mallory could have made those appointments at any time.[25]

* * *

Obtaining the services of competent medical officers in adequate numbers required considerable effort, but surgeons and assistant surgeons alone could not meet all of the medical needs of the CSN. Enlisted men and civilian attendants would be needed to assist medical officers and, in some cases, to provide care when medical officers were not present.

– 5 –

Surgeons' Stewards and Hospital Stewards

Some medical services in the CSN were provided by enlisted men called surgeons' stewards. The USN and CSN also had men called hospital stewards, but the distinction between surgeons' and hospital stewards, especially in the CSN, is not entirely clear. Because USN practices were largely duplicated by the CSN, it is useful to examine the prewar roles of surgeons' and hospital stewards in the USN.

Surgeons' and Hospital Stewards in the Prewar USN

In the 1840s, USN crewmembers who assisted medical officers came to be known as surgeons' stewards. The medical officer on a vessel would select ("rate") a man from the crew to serve in that role. The chosen man, now a petty officer, received more pay than most other sailors, but the selection was not permanent, and a surgeon's steward could be disrated for unsatisfactory performance. Surgeons' stewards performed such tasks as compounding prescriptions, changing dressings, and keeping records. A USN surgeon noted before the war that retaining surgeons' stewards who were competent, sober, and faithful was difficult in the volunteer navy because they were paid so poorly and had no prospect of promotion. A man with those qualities was "certain, on the first opportunity, to engage in any other business which will properly reward him." Instructions issued in 1857 for USN medical officers indicated that hospitals, navy yards, and vessels with a medical officer were entitled to a surgeon's

5. Surgeons' Stewards and Hospital Stewards

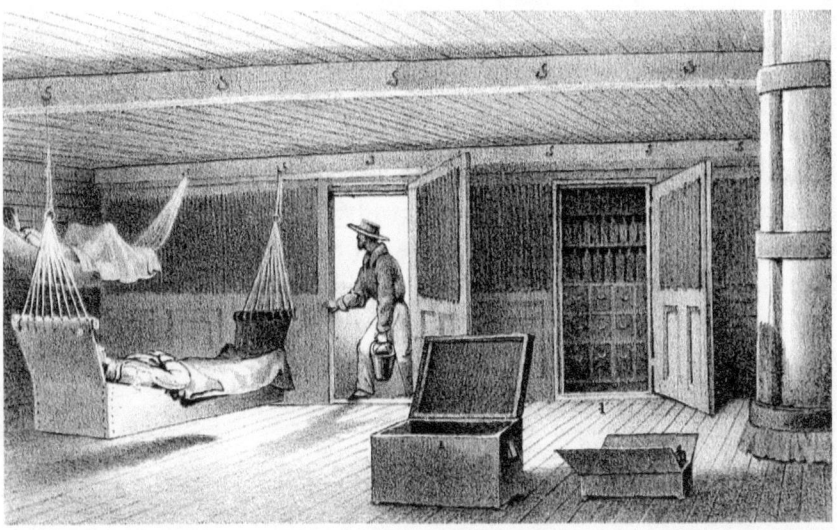

An attendant, possibly a surgeon's steward, entering the sickbay of a USN frigate. The closet encloses the dispensary. On the floor are a chest of surgical instruments and a tray of small articles. Sickbays on most war vessels were probably not this roomy (G.R.B. Horner, *Diseases and Injuries of Seamen*).

steward. In addition to assisting with medical duties, surgeons' stewards may have assumed clerical roles under upper-echelon medical officers such as fleet surgeons or surgeons of station.[1]

Among the civilian employees of naval hospitals was a steward, often called a hospital steward. He was a superintendent, whose duties included supervising other civilian employees—nurses, matrons, cooks, and porters, for example—taking charge of supplies (other than medicines and other medical or surgical articles), purchasing food, keeping certain records, and overseeing the management of the hospital grounds. Assisting with medical care was not among his responsibilities. Because of their civilian status, hospital stewards were absent from lists of naval grades and pay scales. Hospital stewards were, however, paid more than most surgeons' stewards. That situation that led Surgeon William P.C. Barton, chief of the USN's Bureau of Medicine and Surgery, to propose in 1843 to the secretary of the navy that "all stewards for the Medical Department be called surgeon's stewards and that the pay of all be $30 per month.

Good responsible men of competent abilities can not be got for less." Despite Barton's recommendations, both titles still existed in the USN when the Civil War commenced. In 1860, the standard monthly pay for surgeons' stewards was $24, but those serving in navy yards usually received $40 per month; the surgeon's steward at the Mare Island, California, Ship Yard received $62.50 per month. Perhaps certain postings for surgeons' stewards, such as those at navy yards, required more highly skilled men and warranted higher pay. During the same year, hospital stewards received $40 per month.[2]

Surgeons' and Hospital Stewards in the CSN

CSN practices regarding surgeons' and hospital stewards largely mirrored those of the USN. The CSN, for example, had petty officers called surgeons' stewards who served on vessels of war. Early in the war, they were generally paid $24 per month, as opposed to $18 or $16 for seamen and landsmen. (By late 1862, the monthly pay for surgeons' stewards, seamen, and landsmen had risen to $28, $22, and $16, respectively.) Surgeons' stewards were not always selected from men who just happened to enlist as crewmembers. Medical officers—probably surgeons of station or fleet surgeons—sometimes placed advertisements for them and evidently agreed to appoint qualified applicants to that grade once they enlisted in the navy. When Surgeon Lewis W. Minor advertised for a surgeon's steward for CSS *McRae*, he specified, "None need apply who are not accustomed to putting up prescriptions, to keeping accounts, and who cannot write a legible hand."[3]

The CSN also employed hospital stewards, and the omission of that title from lists of grades and pay scales suggests that, as in the USN, hospital stewards were intended to be civilians. Richard Hall, steward at the Richmond Naval Hospital received $40 per month in 1863, as did Robert Wallace at the Savannah Naval Hospital in 1864. John W. Evans received $40 per month in 1863 as steward for the Charleston Naval Hospital, but his pay was increased to $65 per month by early 1864. Hall, Wallace, and Evans all appear to

5. Surgeons' Stewards and Hospital Stewards

have been civilians. The CSN hospital at Smithville, North Carolina, employed W.B. Spikes as an "acting hospital steward." Spikes, whose one recorded action was to buy chairs, chickens, soap, eggs, and vinegar, was probably a civilian acting temporarily as hospital steward.[4]

A booklet of instruction for CSN medical officers (dated November 1, 1862) differed from the 1857 USN version, from which it was modeled, by placing hospital stewards, rather than surgeons' stewards, in navy yards and by omitting surgeons' stewards from the personnel at naval hospitals. Despite the evidence that hospital stewards employed by the CSN were meant to be civilians, that title was sometimes applied to CSN enlisted men. George Morgan, for example, served as a landsman—implying that he had no previous knowledge of the duties of a seaman—on the receiving ship *Dalman* at Mobile Bay before being rated as a hospital steward on February 1, 1863. That change earned him a raise in pay from $16 to $28 per month, a surgeon's steward's usual compensation at the time. John Q.A. Williams was rated as a surgeon's steward at $24 per month in 1862, when he served on CSS *Virginia*. He was then sent to the fortifications at Drewry's Bluff, outside of Richmond, where he was paid $28 per month as a surgeon's steward from October 1862 through late June 1863, after which (through at least March 1864) he was called a hospital steward and paid $40 per month. William Scott, who is listed with military personnel in CSN payrolls, was classified as both a hospital and surgeon's steward and received $40 per month in 1861 and 1862 at the Pensacola Navy Yard.[5]

Perhaps, for enlisted men, the title of surgeon's steward was preferred for duty afloat, which did not apply to receiving ships—on which recruits were processed and trained—or, obviously, to land duty. That possibility, however, does not account for Williams being called a surgeon's steward for his first nine months at Drewry's Bluff or for his pay raise once his title changed from surgeon's steward to hospital steward. Whether Williams's duties changed with his title has not been determined, but it is possible that he had hospital duty at Drewry's Bluff.[6]

Adding to the confusion are examples of the titles of hospital steward and surgeon's steward apparently being used interchangeably. A March 1862 advertisement in a Mobile newspaper advised readers of an opening for a hospital steward—not a surgeon's steward—to serve on the gunboat *Morgan*. That vessel's payroll shows no hospital stewards during that period, but it does include Raphael McBride, formerly rated as a landsman, as a surgeon's steward from early March 1862 through at least the end of the year. John Turner was called a hospital steward when he assisted in keeping medical records on CSS *Atlanta*, a typical task for a surgeon's steward. After that vessel's capture, his grade was recorded by his captors as surgeon's steward, a title appropriate for his being kept in custody to help care for the wounded. A later order to release Turner referred to him as a hospital steward.[7]

It seems likely that formal distinctions between the titles of hospital and surgeon's steward were, at times, ignored, but the mention of both types of steward in the 1862 CSN instruction booklet for medical officers suggests that the titles were not intended to be synonymous. Secretary Mallory mentioned the titles separately in March 1861, when he projected that the CSN's recently acquired facilities at Pensacola would, in keeping with USN practice, require a surgeon's steward at the navy yard and a hospital steward at the associated hospital, each at $40 a month. Mallory also mentioned in 1864 the unconditional release of "naval hospital and surgeons' stewards" who were held prisoner, further implying that the titles were distinct. The naval hospital at Mobile, in fact, employed a hospital steward and surgeon's steward at the same time; they appear, from their position on the payroll, to have been civilians.[8]

It seems safe to conclude that CSN surgeons' stewards were usually enlisted men who served on vessels and that hospital stewards were generally civilians working in naval hospitals. Records, however, are peppered with exceptions to the rule.

Physicians as Surgeons' Stewards

The CSN, at times, offered the position of surgeon's steward to civilian medical practitioners who were to perform the duties of a

5. Surgeons' Stewards and Hospital Stewards

medical officer. As early as December 4, 1861, civilian physician Noah Bennet Benedict was purchasing medical supplies for CSS *Manassas*, indicating his title as "Surgeon, p.t. [pro tempore]." Two weeks later, Flag Officer George N. Hollins at New Orleans ordered Benedict, whom he addressed as an acting surgeon, to duty on *Manassas*. Shortly thereafter, on December 30, Surgeon Lewis W. Minor at the New Orleans Station, with Hollins's approval, appointed Benedict as a surgeon's steward for *Manassas* at a remuneration of $40 and a ration per month. Minor issued similar appointments to civilian physicians John Joseph Steinriede (assigned to CSS *Livingston*) on December 10 and Christopher Columbus Post (assigned to the floating battery *New Orleans*) on January 31. (Steinriede was later appointed as an assistant surgeon for the war.) Minor soon began supplying more specifics in subsequent appointments. He offered a position to Dr. Charles Pelaez on February 12, 1862: "Under authority of the Secretary of the Navy, vested in me, you are hereby appointed Surgeons Steward of the Gun Boat 'Mobile,' at a remuneration of Forty Dollars ($40) pr month and a ration; it being understood that at any time that a Medical Officer shall be appointed to the above named Vessel, thus reducing your pay, or, when you shall desire to leave the service for any other reason or reasons, you shall be discharged so soon thereafter as I can supply your place." Minor used similar language in an offer to Dr. Francis F. Parker, the differences being that Parker was needed on CSS *Manassas* (evidently to replace Surgeon's Steward Benedict), that the appointment of a medical officer to that vessel would reduce Parker's monthly pay to $24, and that Parker was not given the option of leaving the navy.[9]

Benedict, Steinriede, Post, Pelaez, and Parker each signed shipping articles as a seaman or landsman in late 1861 or early 1862 and were quickly rated as surgeons' stewards at $40 per month. Not all surgeons' stewards at New Orleans got the same treatment as the aforementioned physicians. In September 1861, Surgeon Minor advertised in a New Orleans newspaper for a surgeon's steward for CSS *Ivy* at $24 per month and a ration, and Surgeon's Steward Jacob Smith served at the New Orleans station in 1861 and 1862 at a salary of $24 per month.[10]

The Confederate Navy Medical Corps

Although all CSN vessels were supposed to have a surgeon's steward, those with too small a number of crewmembers were not assigned a medical officer. It is unclear whether surgeons and assistant surgeons were planned but too scarce for assignment to CSS *Manassas*, *New Orleans*, and *Mobile* or whether those vessels would ever receive a medical officer. In any case, appointing a physician as a $40-per-month surgeon's steward was a bargain for the navy, because even the least experienced assistant surgeon or civilian contract surgeon would be paid about $104 per month ($1,250 per year) while on sea duty.

The concept of paying selected surgeons' stewards $40 per month probably arose from the USN's practice of offering the same elevated pay (rather than the usual $24 per month) to surgeons' stewards assigned to navy yards. There was no support for doing so in USN or CSN pay scales, but such assignments may have required a higher-than-usual level of skill or responsibility and warranted more substantial remuneration.

* * *

In the CSN, the titles of surgeon's steward and hospital steward were applied inconsistently and, it appears, sometimes interchangeably. Men called surgeons' stewards might be the only providers of medical care on certain vessels and in some cases were physicians. Hospital stewards were traditionally civilians employed in naval hospitals who oversaw the running of the institution without assuming actual patient-care duties. However they were employed, the CSN's surgeons' and hospital stewards were important in providing medical services.

– 6 –

Civilian Physicians

In addition to commissioned medical officers, the CSN employed an undetermined number of civilian physicians without calling them surgeons' or hospital stewards. They can generally be classified as (1) practitioners who saw CSN patients at land-based facilities or visited them on docked vessels, or (2) acting assistant surgeons, who typically served on vessels, usually for the duration of a cruise, and shared the hazards of personnel there assigned. Such civilians may have been assigned by authority of a naval officer or the secretary of the navy, but they were not appointed by the president and were therefore not commissioned, and their names did not appear in official CSN registers. Some civilian physicians who assisted the CSN also did the same for the Confederate army.

Practitioners Staying Local

Local civilian physicians were sometimes hired to care for naval enlisted personnel when a CSN medical officer was not available. In October 1861, James D. Johnston, signing himself as lieutenant in charge at the Mobile Naval Station, informed G. Floyd Johnston that the latter had been appointed "the Medical Officer at this place." Dr. Johnston's first assignment was examining recruits and caring for the crew on the receiving ship *Dalman*. Dr. Johnston evidently did not have an adequate supply of medicines, because during the first quarter of 1862, he was having prescriptions filled, at the navy's expense, by Mobile druggists Buck and Wade. Johnston served for at least six months at $4 per day.[1]

Also employed at a naval station was William H. Hill, M.D.,

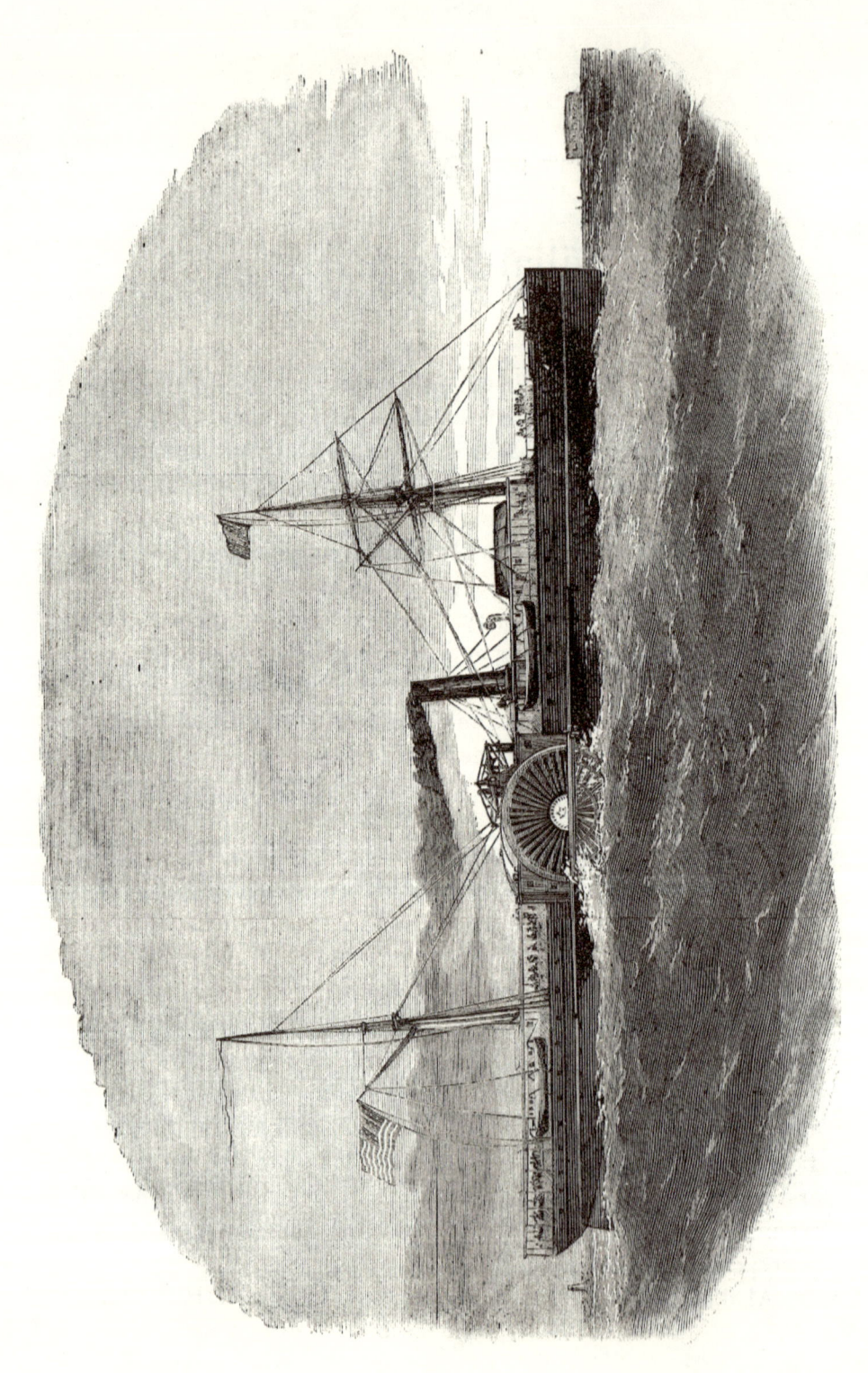

6. Civilian Physicians

who saw patients at Halifax, North Carolina, during parts of 1863 and 1864. His patients included a superintendent, carpenter, clerk, guards, and African American laborers.[2]

Another civilian hired early in the war was Dr. Ralph Darby, who served at New Orleans on the receiving and hospital ship *St. Philip* in May 1861. A newspaper correspondent referred to Darby as "a skillful medical practitioner ... who thoroughly understands the treatment of every ill to which flesh is near." Darby was credited with valiantly diving into the water with life preservers after a boat carrying seven members of *St. Philip*'s crew capsized; four of those crewmembers died in the incident. Darby was also reported to be a medical officer on the cruiser *Sumter*.[3]

In November 1861, Lieutenant Francis E. Shepperd, commanding CSS *Mobile* of the Mississippi River Squadron, wrote that "there being no medical officer on board, was compelled to employ Dr. [A.W.] Goodloe." The physician, apparently based in New Orleans, treated multiple patients on the vessel during October and November, including one for a "private disease." He even traveled to Shell Island—a 15-mile trip for the doctor—to see four sailors manning a launch there. Goodloe also provided contract medical services to the Confederate army.[4]

Dr. F. Hasenburg of New Orleans charged $5 for services rendered to a sailor on CSS *McRae* in 1861, and Dr. John L. Ancrum charged $20 for attending to three sailors at Charleston in 1862. Dr. B.S. Herndon rendered medical and surgical services in December 1861 and January 1862 on CSS *Rappahannock*, which was operating on the Potomac and Rappahannock Rivers, charging $1.50 per patient per day of attendance and services. Carthon Archer, M.D., charged the CSN $633.50 for multiple visits to CSS *Torpedo* on the James River during the first quarter of 1864. His services included

Opposite: Steamer *Star of the West*, which was renamed CSS *St. Philip* after its capture by Confederate forces in April 1861. The vessel was used by the CSN as a hospital and receiving ship at New Orleans, where its medical staff included civilian physician Ralph Darby. *Star of the West* is best known for its use in an unsuccessful Federal attempt to reinforce Fort Sumter in January 1861 (*Harper's Weekly*, Jan. 19, 1861).

providing advice, opening an abscess, furnishing medicines, and vaccinating the crew against smallpox.[5]

Civilian physician F.B. Wakefield saw patients and prescribed medicine in August and September 1862 at Saffold, Georgia, where CSS *Chattahoochee* was being built. It appears that Surgeon Henry W.M. Washington and Assistant Surgeon Marcellus Ford arrived at Saffold shortly thereafter. Some medicines and the "services of a steward" for half a month were evidently procured through the efforts of David S. Johnston, the contractor in charge of constructing the vessel.[6]

Before a CSN hospital was established at Savannah in mid–1863, much use was made of the City Hospital there (also called the Marine or Poor House Hospital). That hospital charged 85 cents a day per patient—50 cents for board, 25 cents for medical attendance by civilian physicians, and 10 cents for medicines. Vessels whose crewmembers were admitted to that facility included CSS *Savannah*, *Huntress*, *Lady Davis*, *Sampson*, *Resolute*, *Fingal*, *Georgia* (floating battery), and *Isondiga*. Although medical officers were probably present on the vessels, there were evidently few or none stationed ashore.[7]

CSN officers who became ill while on duty where no medical officer was present were allowed to be seek care from private physicians and to have the expense reimbursed, "provided said bill shall not exceed the usual charges for similar services at said place." Thus, Lieutenant Wilburn B. Hall, stationed at or near Charleston, received care from Dr. William M. Fitch during four months in 1862 and applied for reimbursement for $44 in medical charges. A naval hospital may not have existed in Charleston at the time, and if Hall required care ashore, rather than on a vessel, his only option may have been to see a civilian doctor.[8]

Acting Assistant Surgeons

Some civilian practitioners, often called acting assistant surgeons, were essentially embedded with officers and men on fighting vessels. Records are unclear about who had the authority to appoint

6. Civilian Physicians

acting assistant surgeons. In December 1861, Surgeon William B. Sinclair of the OMS—possibly filling in for OMS chief Spotswood—informed civilian physician E. Holt Jones that Secretary Mallory had appointed him as a "temporary medical officer." Jones would receive the "pay, rations, and position" of an assistant surgeon and serve as long as Mallory pleased. Jones was with CSS *Seabird* when it was sunk in February 1862 and was paroled shortly thereafter. A similar agreement seems to have been struck with Dr. Archer Hays, who was told in September 1861 by Captain George N. Hollins, commanding at New Orleans, that he had been appointed an acting assistant surgeon. Hays received the pay of an assistant surgeon while serving on CSS *Selma* (originally gunboat *Florida*) in 1862 and was paroled in May 1865; the nature of his intervening service is unclear.[9]

When illness struck both medical officers of CSS *Arkansas*—then on the Mississippi River near Vicksburg and the target of daily shelling from Union mortars—the captain telegraphed an appeal for volunteers. A highly recommended civilian physician (probably Robert Bruce Banks of Clinton, Mississippi) presented himself and was appointed as an acting medical officer.[10] At first, the newcomer seemed delighted with the ship, but he soon exhibited his lack of military bearing. As recounted by an *Arkansas* officer:

> The officer of the powder division started around below to show the new medical officer his station during action, and the arrangements for disposing of the wounded, etc., etc. In going along the berth-deck the officer remarked to the doctor that in a battle there was plenty to do, as the wounded came down in a steady stream. The "medico" looked a little incredulous; but a few minutes afterward, when he perceived the road through which an 11-inch shell had come, his face lengthened perceptibly; and after awhile, when the big shell began to fall around the vessel, he became rather nervous. He would stand on the companion-ladder and watch the smoke rise from the mortar-vessels, and would wait until he heard the whizzing of the shell through the air, when he would make a dive for his state room. As soon as the shell fell he would go up and watch out for another. Occasionally, when a shell would explode close to us, or fall with a heavy splash alongside, he would be heard to groan, "Oh! Louisa and the babes!"[11]

Another civilian physician who helped to treat the wounded on CSS *Arkansas* was one C.R. Henderson of Yazoo County, Mississippi.[12]

The Confederate Navy Medical Corps

Acting assistant surgeons could also be found on commerce raiders. Examples include the aforementioned John L Ancrum on CSS *Nashville*, David Herbert Llewellyn on CSS *Alabama*, and Frederick J. McNulty on CSS *Shenandoah*. Details about Ancrum's appointment have not been found. Llewellyn, an Englishman, was appointed acting assistant surgeon, then acting surgeon, by *Alabama*'s commander, Captain Raphael Semmes, but he was never officially commissioned into the CSN. McNulty was appointed at sea by *Shenandoah*'s commander, Lieutenant James I. Waddell, by virtue of the authority vested in him. That appointment was as acting assistant surgeon, although McNulty claimed after the war that he had been commissioned as an assistant surgeon.[13]

A CSN acting assistant surgeon known only as J.H. Allen, from Virginia, was reportedly captured at Fort Fisher, North Carolina, on January 15, 1865, and released the following May.[14]

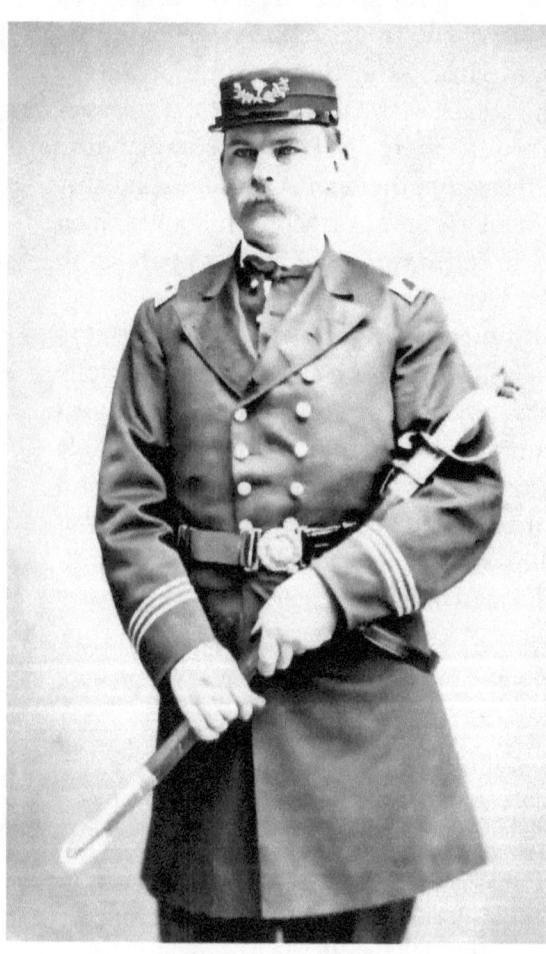

Postwar photograph of Frederick J. McNulty, who served as acting assistant surgeon on the Confederate commerce raider *Shenandoah*. McNulty's uniform may be that of the Chilean navy, in which he served after the American Civil War (courtesy Jonathan O'Neal, M.D.).

6. Civilian Physicians

* * *

How often the CSN had to call on civilian physicians, rather than their own medical officers, is unknown. Using local practitioners rather than commissioned medical officers was probably not preferred because the civilians' competency had not been assessed by examination, they did not necessarily know or abide by naval practice and paperwork, and they were less vulnerable to military discipline. Nevertheless, there were times, particularly early in the war, when medical officers were not where they were needed, and turning to civilian practitioners was the only reasonable option. The CSN did not establish naval hospitals immediately at all sites where naval personnel were numerous, so the use of civilian hospitals and their associated physicians—as in Savannah—was also a reasonable expedient. The manning of Confederate cruisers, if occurring in Europe, might necessitate the assignment of civilians as medical officers. Although much remains unknown about the CSN's use of civilian physicians, those individuals appear to have played a necessary role in supplementing the CSN's roster of commissioned medical officers.

– 7 –

Medical Officers' Assignments

The types of assignments given to CSN medical officers changed as the war progressed and largely reflected the increasing availability of war vessels and shore establishments. Oddly enough, the needs of the Confederate army also came into play, especially early in the war.

The CSN Office of Orders and Detail was responsible for issuing orders regarding assignments on the basis of need as determined by commanders of shore facilities or squadrons, the bureau to which the facilities belonged, the Office of Orders and Detail itself, and Secretary Mallory. When the CSN took control of the ordnance works at Selma, Alabama, for example, the number of men to be assigned there—including one medical officer—were indicated to the facility's commander by the chief of the Office of Ordnance and Hydrography. Those assignments were undoubtedly made in cooperation with the Office of Orders and Detail. The selection of officers and men for certain posts was influenced at times by the wishes of commanders requesting personnel and by the input of the chiefs of various other bureaus of the Navy Department. Surgeon Spotswood, for example, probably provided the Office of Order and Details with the names of medical officers who would be good fits for individual assignments.[1]

In general, the medical officers with the most experience—that is, the oldest—were assigned to shore duty, where they spent most or all of the war. The assignments, for example, of Surgeon James Cornick, who had entered the USN in 1819, appear to have been limited to hospitals and naval rendezvous (recruiting stations). CSN regulations stated that, as a general rule, officers' appointments to shore duty or to receiving ships should continue for two years, subject to

7. Medical Officers' Assignments

the needs of the service. Once a medical officer was ordered to a station or squadron, the commander there could make a more specific assignment.[2]

Changes in postings could be numerous. For example, CSN vessels on which Robert R. Gibbes served—as an assistant surgeon or passed assistant surgeon—included *Lady Davis, Fingal, Savannah, Sampson, Atlanta* (originally *Fingal* before being converted to an ironclad ram), *Georgia, Chicora,* and *Patrick Henry.* He also served at the recruiting office in Savannah and at the Charleston Naval Hospital. Some of the assignments were short and consisted of filling in for an absent medical officer, yet they still represented frequent assignment changes, especially since Gibbes spent about half a year as a prisoner after the capture of CSS *Atlanta.* On June 1, 1864, Gibbes described reporting to Captain Duncan N. Ingraham, commandant of the Charleston Station, to begin his assignment at the naval hospital there. As Gibbes left the building after speaking with Ingraham, a 100-pound shell fired from Union artillerists on Morris Island landed less than six yards away from him but failed to explode. It covered Gibbes with dirt and left him feeling shocked for hours. Observers, especially Ingraham, considered it miraculous that Gibbes had not been injured. Shore assignments were probably presumed to be fairly safe, but Gibbes's experience suggested otherwise.[3]

The CSN's 1864 register of officers provides a good picture of the distribution of assignments given to members of the medical department, with about half assigned to shore duty and half to duty afloat. Twenty-four medical officers, out of 85 included in the register, were shown as assigned to duty ashore (at specified naval stations) but not at a hospital. Such shore duty was most commonly not further described in registers, but specific postings were at various naval rendezvous, on a receiving ship, at an ordnance facility, on the schoolship *Patrick Henry*, or at the OMS. Unspecified shore assignments may also have included naval batteries or vessel-construction sites. The remaining shore assignments were at naval hospitals (10) or at the Drewry's Bluff batteries (3). Two medical officers were awaiting assignment Among the 85 medical officers in the register, slightly more than half (46) were shown as being assigned to a specific vessel or squadron or to "special service" or service abroad, with the last designation meaning service on a cruiser being built in Europe.[4]

Army Assignments

The modest initial needs of the CSN—and evident shortages of experienced medical officers in the Confederate army—triggered the assignment of several CSN surgeons to army duty. William F. Carrington, who filled one of the first five openings for full surgeon in the CSN, was on duty with the OMS in Montgomery by the end of May 1861. By late July 1861, however, he was in Richmond requesting camp supplies from the army quartermaster, and by September 1861, he had been assigned as medical director for General Robert E. Lee's command in western Virginia. Carrington was identified as medical director of the Army of Western Virginia in October 1861 and of the Army of the Northwest in January 1862. In February 1862, he was ordered to inspect a hospital and camp at Fredericksburg; special instructions were to be provided by Surgeon General Samuel Preston Moore of the Confederate army. The next month, Carrington was ordered to conduct similar inspections at Pensacola and Mobile and report his findings to Moore. Payrolls for the Richmond Naval Station from October 1861 through June 1862 show that Carrington signed for his pay. Thus, Carrington was evidently based, at least on paper, in Richmond during that time, and the navy appears to have financed his work for the army. Exactly when Carrington returned to naval duty has not been determined, but he was aboard CSS *Baltic* by December 1862.[5]

Dinwiddie B. Phillips, appointed as a CSN surgeon in June 1861, was assigned in August 1861 as medical director of the forces commanded by Brigadier General Henry A. Wise (Wise's Legion) in western Virginia. Wise evidently contemplated giving Phillips temporary command responsibility, which prompted Phillips to suggest in September 1861 that he be given the temporary grade of lieutenant colonel, since his standing as surgeon and staff officer did not allow him to command. About a week later, Phillips was relieved from his

7. Medical Officers' Assignments

army duties and ordered to report to Secretary Mallory. While serving on CSS *Virginia* (the rebuilt United States ship [USS] *Merrimack*) in March 1862, Phillips asked President Davis to appoint him as major in the army; that request was not granted.[6]

Surgeon Daniel S. Green, who entered the CSN in June 1861, was quickly assigned to duty with the army in Virginia, serving as surgeon in charge of the general hospital at Culpeper Court House from August 1861 until that facility was discontinued March 1862. While there, he was assisted by Assistant Surgeons Bennett W. Green and Marcellus P. Christian, CSN, the latter of whom handled paperwork in September and October 1861 before returning to naval duty in November 1861. Surgeon Green (Daniel S.) subsequently took charge of the army's General Hospital No. 2 in Lynchburg until relieved by an army surgeon in September 1862; for part of that time, he was also surgeon in charge of the army's General Hospital No. 2 in Danville. Like CSN Surgeon Carrington, Surgeon Green was carried on the payroll for the Richmond Naval Station and signed for his pay for October 1861 through June 1862. Surgeon Green returned to naval duty but died in March 1864, after which a group of army surgeons published a tribute to his meritorious official conduct and his "invariably kind and courteous demeanor."[7]

Passed Assistant Surgeon Daniel B. Conrad, USN, had arrived at Boston Harbor on USS *Niagara* in mid–April 1861, after a cruise to Japan. There the crew first heard of the outbreak of war, and the loyalty oath was presented. Conrad, a Virginian, and eight other officers refused to take the oath and were ordered off the vessel. Conrad boarded a train for New York and was arrested by order of Massachusetts governor John A. Andrews. Because he was still an officer in the USN—never having tendered his resignation and not yet dismissed—he was surrendered to naval authorities, who placed him on a naval receiving ship in Boston Harbor. A parole allowed him to go to Boston, where he remained until dismissed from the USN on May 10 for "having refused to take an oath to support the Constitution of the United States." Conrad escaped to New York and eventually made his way to Virginia, where he was commissioned as passed assistant surgeon in the Virginia navy on May 25, 1861. He entered the CSN as a full surgeon on June 6, 1861, and was quickly assigned as surgeon of the Second Virginia Infantry Regiment, with which he served until ordered to naval duty in September 1861.[8]

Conrad's services were requested by the army as late as April 1863, when Surgeon Hunter Holmes McGuire, medical director of the Army of Northern Virginia's Second Corps, asked Secretary of the Navy Mallory to have Conrad ordered to temporary duty with that corps. Although favorably endorsed by corps commander Major General Thomas J. "Stonewall" Jackson, the request was denied.[9]

A newspaper correspondent reported in October 1861 that Assistant Surgeon Algernon S. Garnett, CSN, had organized an army hospital in Dumfries, Virginia, while serving as surgeon of Brigadier General Isaac R. Trimble's Brigade of the Confederate Army of the Potomac. As was the case for CSN surgeon William F. Carrington, Garnett also appeared on the CSN payroll at the Richmond station at that time.[10]

In at least one instance, a CSN medical officer asked that he be allowed to serve with the army late in the war. In September 1864, Surgeon Francis L. Galt, CSN, requested a leave of absence "to join the army for service in the field." Secretary Mallory told Galt that his services were required in the navy and denied the request.[11]

Assignments to Naval Stations, Navy Yards, or Squadrons

The assignments of most CSN medical officers were at shore facilities in the South or aboard vessels that patrolled local waters. Shore facilities included hospitals, naval rendezvous, receiving ships, and storage and repair facilities and were under the overall command of a line officer as the area or station commandant. A station had geographic limits and might include a navy yard, which was particularly involved with docking, repair, and supply and might include manufacturing facilities such as a foundry and sawmill. A navy yard within a station could have its own commandant, distinct from that of its associated station—this was usually the case in the CSN—and could, by itself, constitute a naval station. Station commandants

7. Medical Officers' Assignments

were entitled to a staff that included a surgeon (a surgeon of station). That medical staff officer acted as intermediary between OMS chief Spotswood in Richmond and the medical officers manning the shore facilities. A station commandant might also command the facility's associated squadron, in which case he could also assume the title and additional pay of flag officer. It appears that an officer who commanded both a station and its squadron had a single medical officer on his staff. Limited information suggests that such a medical officer was called a surgeon of station during about the first half of the war and a fleet surgeon thereafter.[12]

Staff surgeons at stations or yards included Surgeon William F. Patton, who served at Charleston and signed himself as "Surgeon of Station," and Surgeon Lewis W. Minor, who served at New Orleans and Mobile and signed as "Surg. C.S.N. Station." Other surgeons of station or yard may have included John W. Sandford, Jr., who signed himself as "Asst. Surgeon & Senior Medical Officer" and later as "Senior Passed Asst. Surgeon" at the Savannah Naval Station; Charles M. Morfit, who signed himself as assistant surgeon at the office of the naval station at Halifax, North Carolina; and Hugh S. Paisley, who signed himself as assistant surgeon in the office of the commandant, Pee Dee Navy Yard, South Carolina. Surgeon William F. Carrington served as "surgeon of the yard" at the Warrington (Pensacola) Navy Yard.[13]

Other medical officers assigned to navy yards or similar facilities included Surgeon Henry W.M. Washington, "Surg'n & Senior Off. in Charge" at Saffold, Georgia; Assistant Surgeon Stephen S. Herrick at the Oven Bluff gunboat construction site on the Tombigbee River, Alabama; Assistant Surgeon Edward Caire at a similar site at McIntosh Bluff, also on the Tombigbee River; and Assistant Surgeons Charles E. Lining and Nathaniel M. Read at Little Rock, Arkansas, where construction work was being conducted on CSS *Pontchartrain*.[14]

The occasional inclusion of *senior* in the titles of medical officers suggests that if a station or yard commandant did not select a surgeon to be on his staff, then the medical officer with the most seniority might assume that title, and its responsibilities, by default.

Surgeon James Cornick, the medical officer with the most seniority in the CSN, was stationed at the Richmond naval rendezvous, but having OMS chief Spotswood based in Richmond evidently obviated the need for a separate surgeon of station at that locale. Requests for changes in medical personnel at a station or navy yard were made by its commandant to the Office of Orders and Detail after consultation with the surgeon of station.[15]

A surgeon of station would not only handle paperwork involving other medical officers at the post, but he also undoubtedly advised the station commandant about how medical personnel could be assigned most optimally. He also recruited civilian employees. While surgeon of station at Mobile in 1863, Surgeon Lewis W. Minor tried to instill a professional atmosphere by issuing general orders dictating the behavior of surgeons' stewards. "When Surgeons' Stewards come into this office," said one order, "they will not speak in loud tones or in familiar language, & will not be seated unless invited to do so. The Surgeon's Steward of this office will see the above order executed." Minor's own steward was expected "to copy immediately on Receipt thereof, all Letters, Circulars, Requisitions, Bills, etc. into the Books provided for those purposes." Furthermore, Minor ordered that his steward "will not leave [the office] between the hours of 8:30 a.m. & 2 p.m. without permission of the Surgeon and then for a Specified period. When sent out on duty, he will return when that duty shall have been performed."[16]

Most assignments afloat were on vessels that were parts of squadrons concerned primarily with local defense. Supervisory medical officers for squadrons (fleet surgeons) performed the same sorts of duties as surgeons of stations—approving and forwarding paperwork, for example—but did so for medical officers assigned to squadron vessels. Fleet surgeons also assisted the medical personnel on the flagship. A fleet surgeon, if serving on the staff of the commander of both a station and squadron, also assumed the usual duties of a surgeon of station. Meanwhile, the squadron commander (flag officer) was responsible, among other duties, for seeing that his vessels were adequately manned. Thus, Surgeon Charles H. Williamson was serving in September 1864 on the flagship *Savannah* as fleet

7. Medical Officers' Assignments

surgeon of the Savannah Squadron commanded by Flag Officer William W. Hunter; the regular medical officer of *Savannah* was Assistant Surgeon Cincinnatus M. Parker. Because of sickness among the squadron's medical officers, including Parker, Williamson had to care for the crews of *Savannah* and of squadron vessels that did not ordinarily have a surgeon. The situation prompted Hunter to request more medical officers from the Office of Orders and Detail, and the chief of that bureau, Captain Sidney Smith Lee fulfilled the orders in the name of Secretary Mallory by assigning two additional medical officers to the squadron.[17]

The position of fleet surgeon appears to have been important enough that the absence of one could prompt the assignment of a temporary substitute. Thus, when Fleet Surgeon William D. Harrison of the James River Squadron was hospitalized in November 1864, the squadron's flag officer, Captain John K. Mitchell, ordered Surgeon Francis L. Galt, stationed at one of the shore batteries on the James River, to report to the flagship, *Virginia II*, and temporarily assume Harrison's duties. A day later, Mitchell, no longer in command of shore batteries, rescinded his order to Galt, and a day after that, Mitchell ordered Surgeon Henry W.M. Washington, then serving on CSS *Fredericksburg*, to remain on that vessel but perform Harrison's duties as fleet surgeon.[18]

The CSN was willing to entertain a proposal from Fleet Surgeons Arthur M. Lynah of the Savannah Squadron and Charles H. Williamson of the Charleston Squadron to switch places. Permission to do so came from the CSN's Office of Orders and Detail, by command of the secretary of the navy, with orders for Williamson to report to Savannah and Lynah to Charleston, both as fleet surgeon. The exchange resulted from formal requests to Richmond from Lynah on February 16, 1864—the same day he reported to Charleston as fleet surgeon—and from Williamson on February 16. Permission was granted quickly, on March 1.[19]

Fleet surgeons other than those mentioned above included Surgeons Daniel S. Green of the James River Squadron, James W.B. Greenhow of the North Carolina Squadron, and Daniel B. Conrad of the Mobile Squadron.[20]

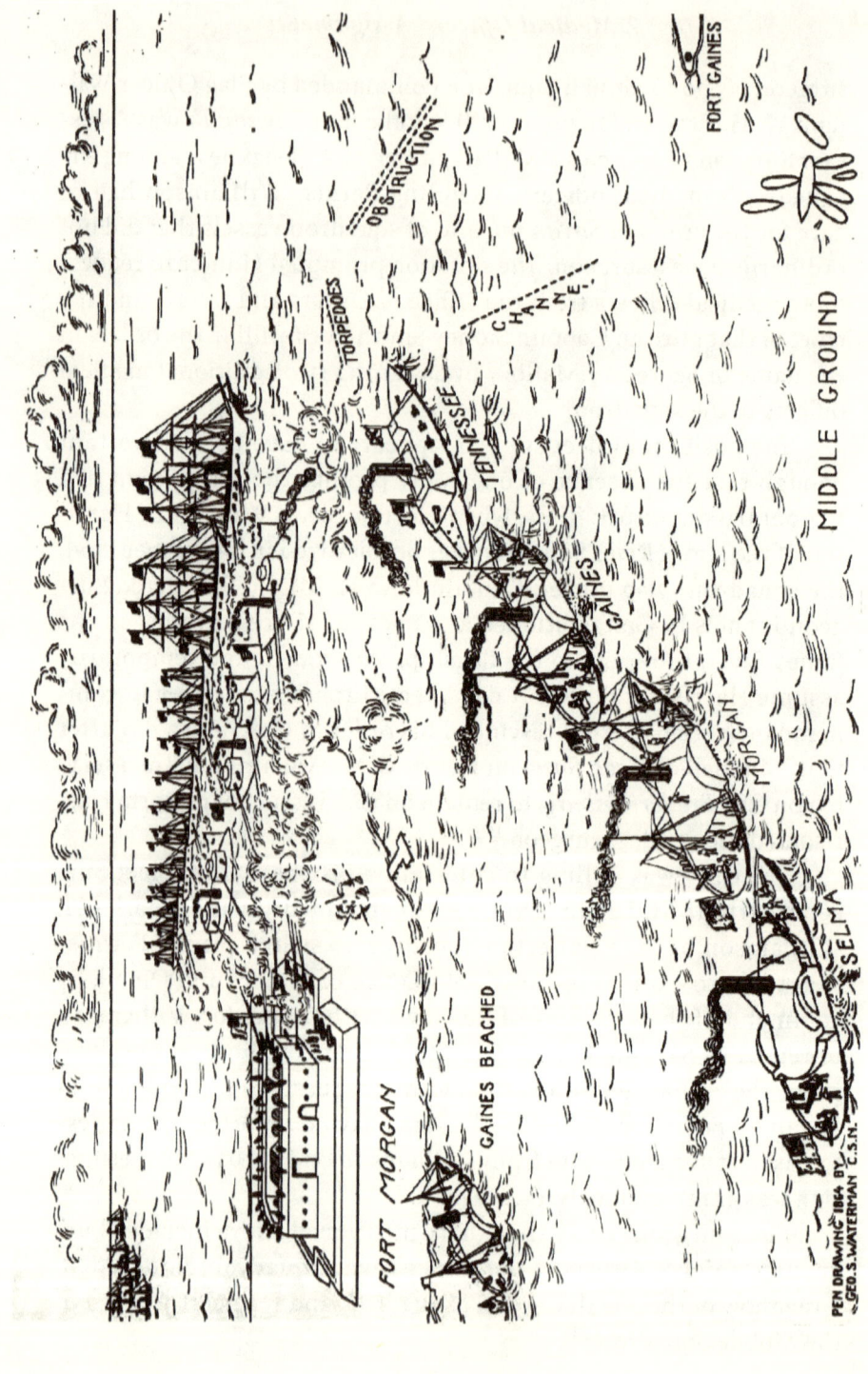

7. Medical Officers' Assignments

Shore Batteries

One common posting for CSN medical officers was with defensive batteries on shore. Among those, the James River batteries, which protected Richmond, probably accounted for the most such assignments. Joining troops from the army and marines in manning the batteries were sailors from the James River Squadron, who operated guns that had been removed from their vessels and mounted at the fortifications; naval surgeons were assigned to care for the marines and sailors.

The most well-known fortification, located about seven miles downriver from Richmond, was at Drewry's Bluff, which was developed to the point of resembling a small village, complete with a hotel, post office, chapel, and soldier-tended market garden. It even served as a terminus for daily pleasure excursions from Richmond on the steamer *A.H. Schultz*. It has not been determined exactly which CSN medical officers were posted to Drewry's Bluff on May 15, 1862, when the guns of the James River fortifications repelled Federal warships threatening Richmond. However, during the war, at least 13 CSN physicians served at Drewry's Bluff, with Surgeon Daniel B. Conrad's assignment lasting about a year and a half. Other medical officers serving there included Surgeons William F. Carrington and Algernon S. Garnett; Passed Assistant Surgeon Charles E. Lining; Assistant Surgeons Pike Brown, Edmund K. Goldsborough, James E. Lindsay, Henry B. Melvin, William Sheppardson, and William Mason Turner; and Assistant Surgeons for the War Edwin G. Booth, Samuel D. Drewry, and Nicholas C. Edmunds. There were reportedly several subterranean hospitals at Drewry's Bluff, but exactly where

Opposite: Ships of the CSN's Mobile Squadron steaming to confront Federal vessels at the Battle of Mobile Bay, August 5, 1864. This southward view shows the squadron's flagship, *Tennessee* (with Fleet Surgeon Daniel B. Conrad and Assistant Surgeon Richard C. Bowles), followed by gunboats *Gaines* (with Passed Assistant Surgeon Osborn S. Iglehart), *Morgan* (probably with Assistant Surgeon Nicholas C. Edmunds), and *Selma* (with Assistant Surgeon Edwin G. Booth). The combined complement of the four CSN vessels was about 470 men (drawing by George S. Waterman, one of *Gaines*'s midshipmen, from his "Notable Events of the Civil War," *Confederate Veteran* 7, no. 1 [Jan. 1899]).

The Confederate Navy Medical Corps

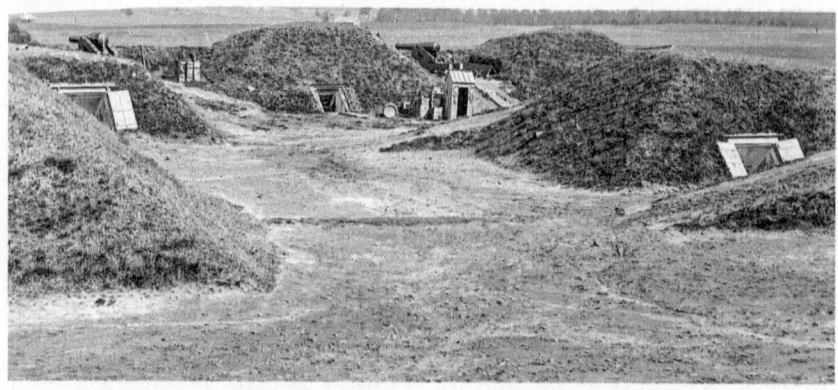

Portion of the Confederate fortifications at Drewry's Bluff, Virginia, several miles downriver from Richmond. The site, which reportedly had underground hospitals, was manned, in part, by CSN personnel, including numerous medical officers (Library of Congress, control no. 2012646744).

naval surgeons were stationed is not clear. At least one ambulance was available, and patients could be transferred to hospitals in Richmond if necessary. Associated fortifications, downriver from Drewry's Bluff, with naval medical officers included Battery Semmes with Assistant Surgeon James G. Boxley and Battery Brooke with Surgeon Francis L. Galt and Assistant Surgeon Richard C. Bowles.[21]

Although assigned to CSS *Patrick Henry* of the James River Squadron, Assistant Surgeon Robert R. Gibbes shuttled among that vessel, the Drewry's Bluff fortifications, and Port Walthall Junction (Virginia) during May 1864 to treat the wounded from clashes with Union troops commanded by Major General Benjamin F. Butler. Gibbes recalled that, for nearly two days, bullets and other projectiles whizzed around him. Left unharmed, the young physician performed seven major operations, probably amputations, and 11 minor ones, such as ligating arteries. Among the men Gibbes treated was a college classmate, who was put aboard CSS *Drewry* for transport to Richmond. There, the patient was admitted to the army's Seabrook Hospital, where he died.[22]

Assistant Surgeon Algernon S. Garnett was stationed at Evansport, Virginia, up to late November 1861. He was evidently assigned

7. Medical Officers' Assignments

to the Cockpit Point batteries along the Potomac River, which had been established early in the war to interfere with commercial shipping to Washington, D.C. Garnett was moved from that assignment to duty on CSS *Virginia*.[23]

Naval surgeons were also assigned to Fort Fisher, which guarded the mouth of the Cape Fear River and thus protected Wilmington, North Carolina. The garrison there when the fort was captured by Union forces on January 15, 1865, consisted of men of the army, navy, and marines. A mile or so from Fort Fisher was Battery Buchanan, whose garrison consisted of sailors from the Wilmington Naval Station, including the North Carolina Squadron. Fort Fisher had a hospital bombproof and at least five army surgeons who were captured. In addition, three naval medical officers—Assistant Surgeons George A. Foote, William W. Griggs, and James M. Hicks—and a naval contract surgeon, J.H. Allen, were taken prisoner when the bastion fell. According to one account, Foote had been ordered to Wilmington and Fort Fisher in late 1864 or early 1865 "and put in charge of hospitals." Assistant Surgeon Hicks was ordered on November 1, 1864, to report to Wilmington "without delay ... for duty in the Naval Battery," but the exact roles that he and other naval surgeons played at Fort Fisher or Battery Buchanan have not been determined.[24]

A Northern newspaper artist, Joseph Becker, who visited Fort Fisher shortly after its capture, described the hospital bombproof, which was located at a crescent battery known as the Pulpit. It contained Confederate troops wounded during the most recent (January) Union bombardment and assault and during an attack the previous month. "Men lay about in the grewsome caverns, with gaping, festering wounds," reported Becker. "The surgeon had been killed, and they got little or no attention until after the fight—a good while after, in fact. Maggots were devouring the flesh of living men. It was too horrible to describe." The identity of the killed surgeon has not been established, but he was apparently not a CSN medical officer.[25]

Officers, men, and guns of CSS *Pontchartrain* were employed at Post of Arkansas (Arkansas Post, Fort Hindman) on the Arkansas River. When Federal forces captured the fort on January 12, 1863,

The Confederate Navy Medical Corps

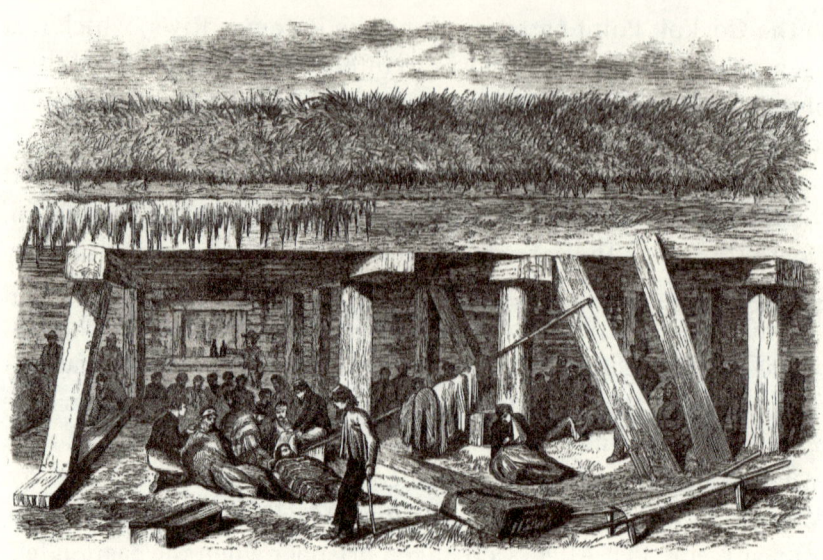

Engraving from Joseph Becker's sketch of the hospital bombproof at Fort Fisher, North Carolina, shortly after the fort's capture by Union forces in January 1865. Confederate naval surgeons may have worked at this site caring for men wounded during the two Union assaults on the bastion (*Frank Leslie's Illustrated Newspaper*, Feb. 18, 1865).

their prisoners included Assistant Surgeon Nathaniel M. Read and more than 30 other naval officers and men. Read's exact role at Post of Arkansas is unknown, but one map of the facility shows that it had a hospital.[26]

At the James River, Fort Fisher, and Arkansas Post batteries, large numbers of men, a fairly sizeable area of defense, and the potential for multiple casualties justified having surgeons present to provide medical care, but at other times, a surgeon was present when smaller batteries were being established. When Midshipman George S. Waterman was directed in 1864 to supervise the construction of a battery guarding Mobile Bay, he was accompanied by Assistant Surgeon William W. Graves and a party of 35 men; they were joined by more than 100 African American workers, who filled sandbags. Waterman and his contingent moved to Battery Buchanan—not to be confused with the fortification of the same name near Fort Fisher—when Federal vessels approached to attack. It is possible that

7. Medical Officers' Assignments

Graves was present not only to care for sick or injured men but to help superintend the work.[27]

When Lieutenant A.F. Warley, CSN, was ordered in July 1861 to set up a battery on the newly occupied Ship Island, off the coast of Mississippi, he landed on the island with guns and other supplies carried on two steamers manned by crewmembers of CSS *McRae*; among the officers were some midshipmen and Surgeon Arthur M. Lynah. Joining Warley's men from *McRae* were 55 marines under Captain R.T. Thom and 75 army infantrymen. While on the island, Warley's battery exchanged fire with USS *Massachusetts*, which withdrew out of range after apparently being struck by a few shots. In his report, Warley praised his colleagues generously. "To Surgeon Lynah, C.S. Navy, I am particularly indebted," wrote Warley. "He was surgeon, soldier, and sailor—everything when an officer was needed—serving more directly under command of Captain Thom." It seems that Lynah's contribution went well beyond providing medical care.[28]

Similar praise was bestowed after the Battle of St. Charles, Arkansas, on June 17, 1862, between Federal vessels ascending the White River and hastily built batteries manned, in part, by Confederate sailors. The defenders obstructed the river by scuttling in it two transports and the gunboat *Maurepas*, whose guns were used in the batteries. The Confederates did great damage to the Union vessels but had to withdraw when approached by Union infantrymen. Among those commended by Lieutenant John W. Dunnington, CSN, who commanded a battery during the battle, was Assistant Surgeon William J. Addison, of *Maurepas*, who "acted with great gallantry, and displayed a coolness and courage unsurpassed by any one in the engagement." Addison's specific feats were not described, but the Confederates sustained only a few casualties before their retreat.[29]

Foreign Service

Although most CSN surgeons assigned to vessels served in home waters, some were sent overseas to serve in ships purchased for the Confederacy in Europe. Most such ships were intended to be commerce raiders and were manned largely by European crews. Surgeon Francis L. Galt, for example, found himself at Gibraltar when his service with the cruiser *Sumter* ended in early 1862. Galt, with that vessel's former commander and executive officer, Raphael Semmes and John M. Kell, traveled to London, Nassau, Liverpool, and finally the Azores to join the new cruiser *Alabama*, which had been built in Liverpool. Lieutenant Arthur Sinclair, Jr., one of *Alabama*'s officers, reported that Galt "did not lose by disease one soul out of the two hundred and thirteen men serving from first to last on the vessel." Galt also served as acting paymaster, and "was as apt at figures as with his instruments and pills." Sinclair declared that Galt could, "upon a pinch ... have performed the duties of a line-officer, having looked on for so many years, with intelligent appreciation, the exigencies and resources of sailor-craft." Indeed, during its losing encounter with USS *Kearsarge* in June 1864, Galt commanded *Alabama*'s magazine and shell-room divisions while Acting Surgeon David Herbert Llewellyn treated the wounded, and as *Alabama* sank, Galt took charge of a boat that transported injured sailors to *Kearsarge*.[30]

Passed Assistant Surgeons Thomas J. Charlton, Jr., and Bennett W. Green were among a group of officers ordered in May 1863 from Charleston to Bermuda on CSS *Robert E. Lee* (formerly *Giraffe*) and from there to Europe. In February 1864, Charlton and Assistant Surgeon Thomas Emory joined the Liverpool-built cruiser *Florida* at Brest, France. Green was assigned to the cruiser *Rappahannock* at Calais in September 1864 and to the ironclad ram *Stonewall* in January 1865. *Rappahannock*, built in England, docked at Calais for repairs and never served during the war, while *Stonewall*, built in France, never engaged in battle. Other medical officers in Europe included Passed Assistant Surgeon James W. Herty, assigned to CSS *Stonewall*; Passed Assistant Surgeon James E. Lindsay, ordered to be ready to report to *Rappahannock*; Passed Assistant Surgeons Charles E. Lining, who served on CSS *Shenandoah*; and Assistant Surgeon Thomas J. Wheeden, whose assignment has not been determined.[31]

7. Medical Officers' Assignments

* * *

Medical officers in the CSN, especially the younger ones, could expect a fairly wide variety of responsibilities during their wartime experiences. Assignment to a war vessel promised many mundane tasks but came with the potential for exciting and dangerous action. Shore assignments could be fairly sedate, as in the case of naval rendezvous or hospitals. They might also entail combat operations, as with shore batteries, and the risk of injury or capture.

– 8 –

Surgeons Afloat

Physicians who served on CSN vessels left relatively little written description of their medical activities. However, because many CSN officers had served in the USN, their customs and practices presumably continued to a large extent on Confederate vessels. Thus, accounts of how things were done on USN vessels probably describe with fair accuracy how their Confederate counterparts functioned during the war.

A USN surgeon wrote in 1854 that ships of the line, frigates, and sloops were entitled to a full surgeon. Furthermore, a ship of the line was entitled to two additional (lower ranking) medical officers, a frigate to one, and a sloop to none. Vessels smaller than a sloop were not entitled to a full surgeon but could have one passed assistant surgeon or assistant surgeon. CSN regulations stated that the Navy Department would, from time to time, create a table that "shall regulate the number and class of officers, seamen, and other who shall constitute the complement of each class of vessel." Those regulations stated that vessels with a complement of more than 200 men should be commanded by a captain, those with 75–200 men by a commander, and those with smaller complements by a lieutenant. However, no document showing the appropriate number of CSN medical officers per vessel has been found. The Confederate Navy Department evidently contemplated requiring that ironclad vessels should have full surgeon, a consideration that influenced the recommendations made by OMS chief Spotswood about how many officers of that grade were needed.[1]

The medical staffing of a vessel might depend on its expected action. When Surgeon Henry W.M. Washington of the ironclad *Fredericksburg* of the James River Squadron became ill in May 1864

8. Surgeons Afloat

and was hospitalized, that vessel was left with only one medical officer. Squadron Commander John K. Mitchell consequently assigned Assistant Surgeon William J. Addison of CSS *Patrick Henry*—which was used as the base of the Confederate Naval Academy and had two medical officers—to CSS *Fredericksburg* for temporary duty, because he deemed it "essential that she [*Fredericksburg*] should be provided with two medical officers at this time." Mitchell was anticipating *Fredericksburg* and other squadron vessels moving downstream to do battle with Federal vessels moving toward Richmond.[2]

In addition to a surgeon's steward, the largest CSN vessels usually had two medical officers—typically a surgeon or passed assistant surgeon and an assistant surgeon—while smaller vessels might have just one passed assistant surgeon or assistant surgeon. Some CSN vessels had a surgeon's steward only and no medical officer. For most of July 1864, CSS *Palmetto State* had three medical officers: Passed Assistant Surgeon Robert J. Freeman and Assistant Surgeons John P. Lipscomb and Walter E. Bondurant.[3]

Even when not in battle, the surgeon's job was to see to the well-being of the crew (Appendix B). He was to examine men when they joined the ship's crew, promote the acquisition and proper storage of healthful food and clean water, and advise the commander about minimizing outbreaks of infectious diseases—by not anchoring, for example, in marshy areas thought to engender malaria. Because ventilation was notoriously poor in lower sections of the ship, one of the most beneficial suggestions a surgeon could offer was to employ wind sails—large canvas tubes held open by interior hoops, with one end open to the wind and the other directing the fresh air into the damp, hot, and malodorous spaces below. CSN surgeons recognized that the intolerably warm interior of ironclads was unhealthful and recommended that, when such vessels were anchored, crews be permitted to make their quarters on canal boats or other craft or to stay in tents on shore.[4]

Among the healthful activities recommended by surgeons was "bathing in fresh or sea water ... whenever it be of moderate temperature." One option, especially for inexpert swimmers, was to bathe on a beach. Thus, in May 1863, cruiser *Florida*, then off the coast of

Brazil, sent several officers, including Passed Assistant Surgeon Joseph D. Grafton, Jr., ashore in a boat so they could bathe. The boat was upset while crossing a bar, and Grafton drowned after giving up an oar, which he was grasping to keep afloat, to a man who could not swim.[5]

Paperwork could be considerable. Medical officers were responsible for preparing requisitions and receipts for supplies, bills charged against the medical department, and annual returns showing property on hand, receipts, and expenditures. They kept a register showing when and why patients were admitted to sickbay and when they were discharged. They made a quarterly report of sick and expenses, with the latter including a calculated average daily cost per man. For reporting disease and injuries, surgeons were to use a standardized nomenclature of medical terms (in Latin), which would presumably help the OMS tabulate navy-wide health statistics. Separate forms were completed for deaths and cases of disability. A journal of daily practice—typically showing the names and treatments of patients—was to be maintained, as was a notebook, which would record "such matters of interest as may come under his [the surgeon's] notice in relation to climate, disease, medical statistics, and any other professional matter."[6]

Naval surgeons could also be assigned as-needed tasks. After a number of officers on CSS *Atlanta* had been detached from the vessel, for example, Assistant Surgeon Robert R. Gibbes was assigned as a watch officer, a responsibility not ordinarily given to staff officers.[7]

Sickbay

Crewmembers with minor medical complaints could be seen and treated when they presented themselves to a medical officer, while patients whose ailments, in the opinion of that officer, should excuse them from regular duty, would be included in a daily detailed report for the commander. Another list, the so-called binnacle list, consisted of names and grades only and was typically prepared by an assistant surgeon or steward and left at the ship's binnacle (the

8. Surgeons Afloat

housing for the compass). The ship's officers would then know who had been excused from duty and who, according to the surgeon's instructions, should not receive his spirit ration that day. The medical officer would typically see patients in the morning to prescribe for them and visit again in the evening. An assistant, often a surgeon's steward, usually saw the patients at other times of the day and attended to other medical duties, such as preparing medications, changing dressings, and keeping records.[8]

Disagreements related to the sick list could arise. According to Surgeon G.R.B. Horner, USN:

> Some [persons] are for being put on it without being fit subjects for treatment; others object to being left off the list, when deemed well by the medical officers; and a third set object to being put on it at the same time that they want and apply for medicines. A fourth set desire to be reported as sick and excused from duty, but wish to treat themselves, or to be treated by the assistant surgeons instead of the surgeon, or by one of another ship, or, if in port, by private physicians.... From time to time also disputes arise about retaining invalids on the sick list contrary to the wishes of the commander or other officers. At other times men get on the list by feigning indisposition to save themselves from punishment, or to skulk from duty.[9]

On smaller vessels, which might not have a space set aside as the sickbay—also called the ship's hospital—patients were placed wherever convenient. In almost all cases, regardless of the presence of a dedicated sickbay, patients were kept on the berth deck, the level on which crewmembers slept. A patient could occupy his regular sleeping place or be put in a suspended cot nearby, with the displaced sailor taking the patient's previous spot. Dedicated sickbays might have space for a few cots and adjoin a dispensary, where medical supplies were stored and medications could be prepared. Despite physicians' belief that patients needed plenty of air space and ample ventilation, sickbays were almost always poorly ventilated. They were usually poorly lit and could be unbearably warm, especially in an ironclad or if close to a steamer's furnaces or to galleys, where food was prepared. If the sickbay did not have an overhead hatch, and a severely ill or injured sailor needed care during sleeping hours, it was "necessary to drag him ... beneath the hammocks of the crew to get him to the hospital." This was "difficult and painful to him and carriers, from the hammocks being hung only a few feet above the deck, and obliging the latter to stoop very low while they drag the former."[10]

If circumstances allowed, patients with a contagious disease or in need of more care than could be provided aboard could be transferred to a naval or civilian hospital ashore or to a hospital ship. The need for transfer could take time to become apparent. On December 8, 1861, Fireman Oscar Ferris was admitted to the sickbay of CSS *General Polk*, which was stationed on the Mississippi River near Columbus, Kentucky. Ferris initially appeared to have an ordinary case of malaria, but he soon developed pleurisy, became much more ill, and was transferred on December 14 to an army hospital. Ferris died at the hospital on December 18. Ordinary Seaman John Walters was admitted to the sickbay of CSS *Gaines* of the Mobile Squadron on August 14, 1862, with diarrhea, did not improve, and was transferred to a hospital two weeks later. In contrast, Ordinary Seaman Nicholas Halford, admitted to the same sickbay on October 3, 1862, with malaria and cough, was quickly recognized as needing more intensive care and was transferred to a hospital ashore the next day.[11]

Transfer ashore could even involve patients staying at private homes. Assistant Surgeon Osborn S. Iglehart of CSS *Gaines* admitted Midshipman E. Harleston Edwards to sickbay on August 17, 1863, with malaria. Edwards was transferred to a hospital in Mobile on August 22 "to recover his strength," and on August 23, he was sent to a private residence. On August 24, Iglehart was called to see the patient, whose condition had worsened. Iglehart consulted with a civilian physician and visited Edwards at least three more times before the midshipman died on August 27. Between those visits, Iglehart continued seeing patients on CSS *Gaines*.[12]

Because of the limited care and space available on vessels, sickbay patients tended to be those who were judged likely to return to duty within a short time. Among the 973 sickbay admissions for seven vessels in the Savannah Squadron during the first three quarters of 1863, for example, only six patients died. During the same period, the Savannah Naval Hospital recorded 128 admissions and

8. Surgeons Afloat

four deaths. Vessels could also care for patients from other naval facilities. A number of patients were sent from the receiving ship *Savannah*, at Savannah, to ironclad *Atlanta*, stationed nearby off Fort Jackson. They were later "transferred back to the *Savannah* where they can have good quarters and suitable diet."[13]

A patient who no longer required hospitalization aboard but was thought unable to perform useful service in the future was considered for discharge from the navy. That outcome required a "survey" by a board of medical officers—for vessels at sea, surgeons from other ships in the squadron were involved—to examine the patient and determine his degree of disability. Thus, on November 20, 1862, five men of CSS *Gaines* were discharged, having been "condemned" by a medical survey. Records kept on CSS *Gaines* noted that the sailors' diseases were determined not to have originated in the line of duty, a judgment that would affect the ability of those men to collect a pension.[14]

The number of patients on the binnacle list could vary dramatically, as illustrated by sickbay records kept on CSS *Gaines*, which had a reported complement of 130 officers and men. During three days in late December 1862 and early January 1863, the vessel had no sickbay patients, whereas it had 29 patients on August 28, 1863, when malaria was prevalent. The average patient count on CSS *Gaines* was about 1.3 in December 1862 and 19.5 in August 1863. In fact, Flag Officer Franklin Buchanan of the Mobile Squadron reported in August 1863 that 182 of his men were in sickbays or at the naval hospital. The unavailability of the ill, along with losses caused by death, desertion, or discharge (because of disability), resulted in his squadron's vessels being "scarcely half manned." In August 1864, Flag Officer John K. Mitchell of the James River Squadron reported that about a third of the men in his command were sick.[15]

Medical officers were not free from the risk of illness. Among the sick in Mitchell's command in November 1864 were Assistant Surgeon James G. Boxley, assigned to Battery Semmes (one of the James River fortifications), Assistant Surgeon Edmund K. Goldsborough of CSS *Fredericksburg*, and Fleet Surgeon William D. Harrison, all of whom were sent to the Richmond Naval Hospital. Of nine medical officers assigned to the Savannah Squadron in late September 1864, two had been admitted to the Savannah Naval Hospital, two were on sick leave, two had not yet reported for duty, and three were well and on duty. Assistant Surgeon David E. Ewart, assigned to CSS *Chicora* of the Charleston Squadron, died in October 1864 of yellow fever at the Charleston Naval Hospital.[16]

Battle Stations

A surgeon's preparation for battle actually began before his vessel left port, for he was responsible for seeing that the ship had an adequate supply of medical stores and that they were placed where they could be conveniently retrieved. Other medical officers assigned to the vessel, the surgeon's steward, and designated crewmembers were under the surgeon's charge during battle, and they required instruction and rehearsal to ensure that they could perform their assigned roles in an emergency.

In anticipation of combat, the surgeon and his assistants would ready the area of the ship designated by the commander to receive the wounded. That area was often the cockpit, where the officers' quarters and ward room were located, but could be elsewhere in a relatively shielded portion of the vessel. Sick patients resting in the sickbay or elsewhere were relocated to the cockpit or to some other relatively safe place in the vessel, and the dispensary's medicine bottles were moved "to guard against the chance of fragments of glass, and corrosive or inflammable liquids being driven about by the enemy's shot." The risk of such damage was real. A shot striking CSS *Arkansas* "passed through the port-side into the dispensary, mashed up all the drugs, etc., carried in an ugly lot of iron fragments and splinters, passed over the engine-room, grazed the steam-chimney, and lodged in the opposite side of the ship." It killed or injured several crewmembers. Enemy gunfire was not necessary for such damage to occur. Assistant Surgeon Robert J. Freeman, medical officer of CSS *General Polk*, reported that on March 6, 1862, at New Madrid, Missouri, the concussion from one of the vessel's own guns broke

8. Surgeons Afloat

some medicine bottles stored in the dispensary and resulted in their contents being lost.[17]

Tasks for the medical officers and their assistants included clearing the receiving area of unnecessary articles, setting up a platform for surgery—often the table in the ward room ordinarily used for dining—and ensuring that water, medicines, and other supplies were handy. Amputation saws, scalpels, bullet forceps, clamps, and other surgical instruments were laid out ready for use. Basins, buckets, and mops were positioned, as was a supply of sand to sprinkle on the wet or bloodied deck for sure footing. The surgeon was also responsible for distributing tourniquets—bandages and other emergency supplies might also be furnished—to various crewmembers who had previously been instructed about their use. Once preparations were complete, the surgeon informed the executive officer of that fact and stood by to receive patients. An officer of CSS *Arkansas* described battle preparations on the ironclad ram: "The decks were sprinkled with sand and tourniquets and bandages at hand ... down in the berth deck were the surgeons with their bright instruments, stimulants and lint."[18]

As patients arrived, the surgeon prioritized their treatment such that those with serious but apparently survivable injuries, especially with active hemorrhage, were attended to first. Patients with injuries thought to be fatal might be given an opiate or chloroform to reduce pain and moved out of the way, while those who were clinically stable had to wait their turn. In case of fire, the surgeon and his assistants were to be prepared to dispose of any inflammable medical supplies that might feed the blaze and to direct the removal of patients. Probably the most dangerous medical item in the presence of flames was ether, which was highly volatile and inflammable. In fact, if care was to be rendered under the light of lanterns—during battle or not—surgeons would probably keep their stores of ether elsewhere and instead use chloroform as an anesthetic.[19]

Vessels without medical officers made their own preparations. Lieutenant William H. Parker, commanding CSS *Beaufort*, one of the small vessels of the "Mosquito Fleet" operating in the sounds of North Carolina, watched crewmembers preparing bandages by

The Confederate Navy Medical Corps

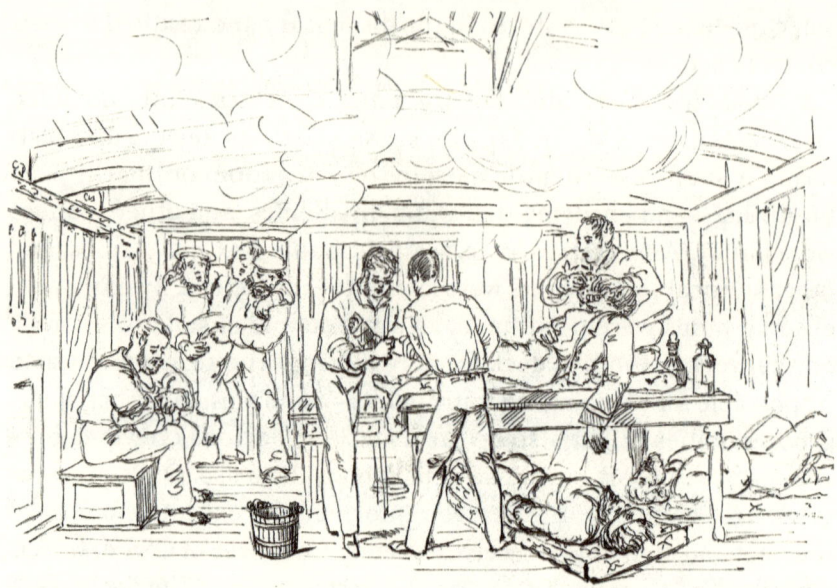

Sketch by Charles Ellery Stedman of medical care being rendered in the cockpit of a Civil War naval vessel during or after battle. The assistant at the patient's head is probably administering chloroform (Civil War Photograph Collection, vol. 14, MOLLUS-MASS, USAHEC).

tearing sheets. "It was one of the delights of serving in these gunboats that no surgeons were allowed," he recalled wryly. "All the wounded had to be sent to the flagship for treatment."[20]

Crewmembers carried their wounded comrades to the cockpit for treatment. Some vessels were equipped with special cots or litters designed to assist in lowering wounded sailors to the cockpit's deck. During the Battle of Mobile Bay on August 5, 1864, Surgeon Daniel B. Conrad of the ironclad ram *Tennessee* was told that Flag Officer Franklin Buchanan, who was topside, had been wounded. Conrad went up himself, found the admiral seriously wounded in the leg, and carried him down to the cockpit himself. Buchanan commended Conrad for his "skill, promptness, and attention to the wounded" during the battle.[21]

The admiral had been struck by a fragment of iron from a shell or from *Tennessee*'s armor. During the battle, in which the combatant vessels sometimes touched, Conrad also attended to gunshot

8. Surgeons Afloat

wounds and to "unburnt cubes of cannon powder" that had "perforated the flesh and made these great blue ridges under the skin." Conrad reported those blue elevations as extremely painful but of no lasting harm. Two crewmembers were leaning against an armor shield when that structure was evidently struck by an enemy shot. "At the same instant," said Conrad, "the men were split into pieces. I saw their limbs and chests, severed and mangled, scattered about the deck, their hearts lying near their bodies." Hits from enemy fire could spray deadly wood splinters, as Conrad observed when taken aboard USS *Hartford* after the battle. There he saw "a long line of grim corpses dressed in blue, lying side by side ... two whole gun's crews ... all killed by splinters." When a *Hartford* officer pointed "to a piece of weather-boarding ten feet long and four inches wide," Conrad gained his "first and vivid idea of what a splinter was."[22]

Passed Assistant Surgeon Osborn S. Iglehart also saw the effect of splinters on crewmen of CSS *Gaines* during the Battle of Mobile Bay. A splinter killed a seaman by ripping open his abdomen, leaving the "contents entirely exposed," and another splinter badly lacerated the fingers of a landsman, although he survived and did not require amputation. An exploding shell killed another sailor by also tearing open his abdomen, "the intestines escaping through the wound," while "fracturing and terribly lacerating his right thigh." Yet another shell inflicted severe contusions on the legs of a seaman, who survived the battle. Iglehart was cited, among other men, for his "coolness and gallantry ... and for the influence it [his deportment] must have had among the crew, most of whom had never before been in action."[23]

Although CSN statistics on surgery are unavailable, Iglehart's descriptions suggest that surgeons performed amputation, and perhaps other major procedures, on ships. Amputation would have been carried out as quickly as practicable after occurrence of the injury, with chloroform or ether, if available, used as an anesthetic. Patients who had undergone amputation would probably be transferred ashore at the earliest convenient opportunity. Amputation was sometimes needed after shipboard accidents not related to combat.[24]

Iglehart was among many medical officers whose behavior in battle afloat was praised. According to Flag Officer Franklin

The Confederate Navy Medical Corps

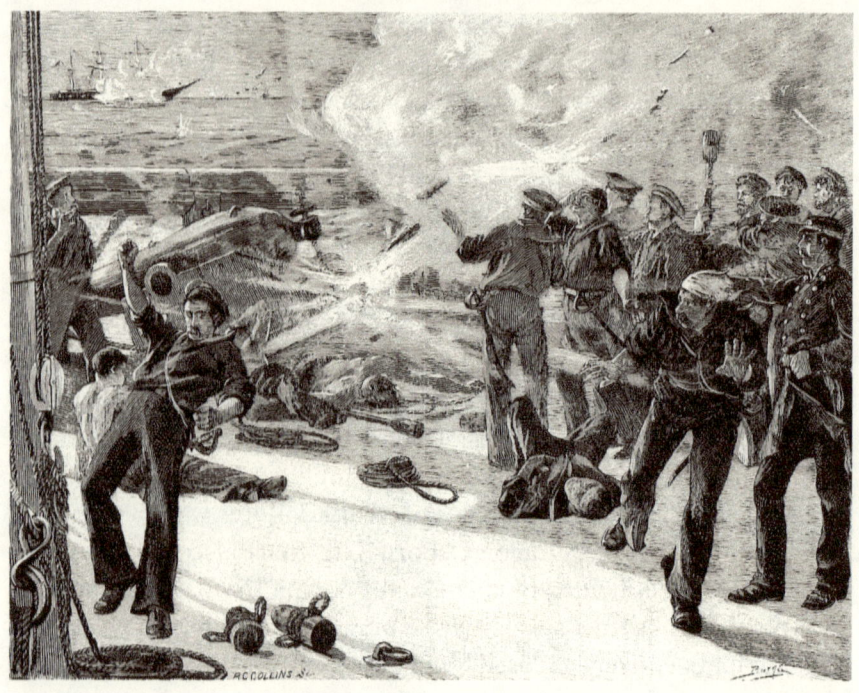

An 11-inch shell from USS *Kearsarge* striking CSS *Alabama* during their June 19, 1864, battle near Cherbourg, France. *Alabama*, which was sunk, had nine men killed, 10 drowned, and 21 wounded out of a complement of about 145. Injuries were caused not only by shell fragments but also by wood or metal splinters (illustration by M.J. Burns in Kell, "Cruise and Combats of the 'Alabama'").

Buchanan, aboard CSS *Virginia* during the March 1862 Battle of Hampton Roads, Surgeon Dinwiddie B. Phillips and Assistant Surgeon Algernon S. Garnett "were prompt and attentive" in performing their duties and earned the gratitude of the wounded by their skillful treatment. Garnett, who was first in line for promotion to full surgeon, earned Buchanan's endorsement for that advancement. Lieutenant Charles W. Read commended Passed Assistant Surgeon Marcellus P. Christian for his prompt attention to the wounded aboard CSS *McRae* during action near Forts Jackson and St. Philip, Louisiana. Assistant Surgeon C. Wesley Thomas earned the respect of Assistant Surgeon W.H. Pierson, USN, of USS *Water Witch*, which was captured by a Confederate boarding party. Thomas, who helped

8. Surgeons Afloat

treat the wounded on *Water Witch*, was praised by Pierson as "an honorable and gentlemanly adversary."[25]

Less serious battle injuries, as reported in surgeons' journals, included lacerations from a sword, treated by Assistant Surgeon Robert J. Freeman of CSS *General Polk*, and a laceration from "a blow from the end of a musket," treated by Freeman and Assistant Surgeon Robert R. Gibbes of CSS *Atlanta*. Those officers, when serving aboard *Atlanta*, treated two gunshot wounds between December 1862 and June 1863, both of which had resulted from accidental discharges of weapons.[26]

The only Confederate naval physician known to have died as a result of battle was Englishman David Herbert Llewellyn, acting surgeon of the cruiser *Alabama*. In June 1864, *Alabama* was defeated in battle by USS *Kearsarge* off the coast of Cherbourg, France. As *Alabama*'s executive officer was assessing damage to the vessel, he saw Llewellyn "at his post" in the wardroom, "but the table and the patient upon it were swept away from him by an eleven-inch shell, which opened in the side of the ship an aperture that was fast filling the ship with water." Llewellyn reportedly assisted in transferring patients to the care of the *Kearsarge*'s surgeons, and he drowned as *Alabama* sank.[27]

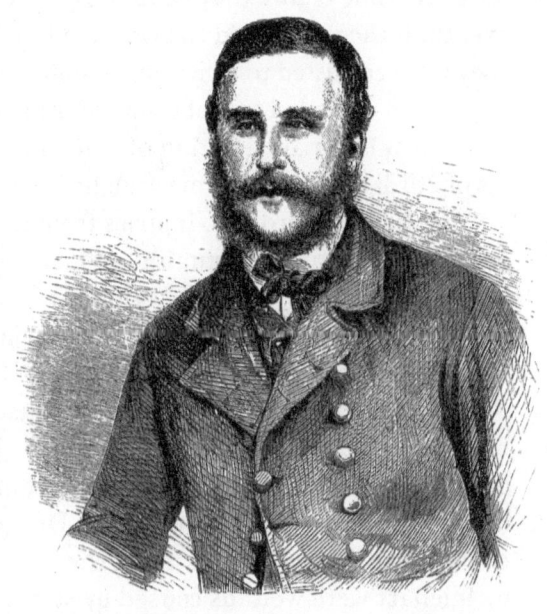

David Herbert Llewellyn, who was appointed as acting surgeon on CSS *Alabama* by its commander, Captain Raphael Semmes. Llewellyn drowned as *Alabama* sank after its battle with USS *Kearsarge* (Kell, "Cruise and Combats of the 'Alabama,'" from a portrait in the *Illustrated London News*, July 8, 1864).

Nonbattle Injuries

Battle was not the only event that could injure large numbers of sailors. On May 27, 1863, the boiler of the gunboat *Chattahoochee* exploded while the vessel was on the Apalachicola River in the Florida panhandle. A dozen or so men were killed immediately. Assistant Surgeon Marcellus Ford, the only medical officer aboard, was knocked down and scalded but recovered sufficiently and "exerted every effort to relieve the sufferings of the wounded." Men were "running about frantic with pain, leaving the impression of their bleeding feet, and sometimes the entire flesh, the nails and all, remain behind them." The wounded were moved to the river bank, but because of a raging storm, "the poor fellows lay writhing and groaning in the mud for some time before they could be got to a cotton gin near by." Ford eventually accompanied the wounded to Columbus, Georgia, where they were admitted to a civilian hospital. The weather that hampered care of the wounded probably had nothing to do with the boiler explosion but was a manifestation of "the only landfalling hurricane now [as of 2013] recorded in American history in the month of May."[28]

Sailors were prone to injuries from the normal activities of shipboard life. Contusions, sprains, and lacerations were fairly common. Ordinary Seaman Michael Maloney of CSS *Atlanta* suffered a partial dislocation when his elbow became jammed between a gun and its port. Assistant Surgeon Iglehart of CSS *Gaines* treated Seaman Francisco Sabarino for a contusion caused by being "struck in the breast by a heavy log," Seaman Dominic Levin for a wound caused by having a nail driven into his foot, Seaman M.S. Hynde for a hand lacerated by glass, and Seaman John Durano for a wound to the head caused by an iron poker. Among the most unexpected injuries seen by Iglehart were wounds caused by stingray attacks (in three different men) and catfish spines (in at least one man, but probably two).[29]

Medical officers were not immune to injury. Assistant Surgeon Robert R. Gibbes became faint during the early stages of dysentery, fell about 12 feet down an open hatch, and sustained severe contusions to his head and shoulder. He wondered why the tumble had not killed him instantly.[30]

8. Surgeons Afloat

Capture

Accounts of Confederate medical officers being injured while serving afloat are rare, but like their colleagues assigned to shore batteries, they ran the risk of being captured. At least 12 commissioned medical officers and one contract surgeon were taken prisoner when their vessels were sunk, captured, or abandoned. One assistant surgeon, Joseph S. Tipton, was captured twice—with the surrender of CSS *Bombshell* and CSS *Resolute*—despite serving for less than half of the war. Others taken prisoner included Assistant Surgeon Edwin G. Booth (with CSS *Selma*), Surgeon Daniel B. Conrad and Assistant Surgeon Richard C. Bowles (with CSS *Tennessee*), Passed Assistant Surgeon Thomas J. Charlton, Jr., and Assistant Surgeon Thomas Emory (with CSS *Florida*), Passed Assistant Surgeon Robert J. Freeman and Assistant Surgeon Robert R. Gibbes (with CSS *Atlanta*), Surgeon Francis L. Galt (with CSS *Alabama*), Assistant Surgeon Joseph D. Grafton, Jr. (with CSS *Louisiana*), Surgeon James W.B. Greenhow and contract surgeon E. Holt Jones (with CSS *Seabird*), and Assistant Surgeon Charles M. Morfit (with CSS *Oconee*). Shortly after his December 1863 return to the South, Gibbes published unsigned accounts of the loss of the *Atlanta* and his imprisonment of several months.[31]

Officers and men captured by the USN were typically transferred to the custody of the U.S. Army when convenient. How Federal officials handled prisoners of war was influenced by military and political considerations—including how the Confederates treated Union prisoners—and changed throughout the war. In early June 1862, the U.S. War Department declared, "The principle being recognized that Medical Officers should not be held as prisoners of war, it is hereby directed that all Medical Officers so held by the United States shall be immediately and unconditionally discharged." That order prompted the immediate release of CSN Assistant Surgeon Grafton, who had been captured near New Orleans in late April 1862 and imprisoned at Fort Warren in Boston Harbor. In an August 1864 letter to U.S. secretary of the navy Gideon Welles, Rear Admiral David G. Farragut, USN, expressed his understanding that "the rebels ... refuse to exchange our Navy officers except for Navy officers." Furthermore, said Farragut, the U.S. held three CSN surgeons (Booth, Bowles, and Conrad), "but I am not advised as to the course pursued by our enemies with this class of officers." After Conrad was released, by late October 1862, he was informed by Secretary Mallory that "all surgeons are now unconditionally released by both sides; none are now held by either. This is the present understanding, and we now hold none as prisoners of war." That understanding evidently did not apply through the rest of the war.[32]

Capture and release dates are not available for all CSN surgeons taken prisoner, but it appears that their length of confinement could last from a day or two to several months. Many captive surgeons were granted parole by promising in writing that, until duly exchanged, they would not take up arms or serve against the U.S. or divulge anything to the detriment of the U.S. that they may have heard in captivity. In some cases, surgeons had their confinement prolonged by volunteering or being assigned to help care for their sick or wounded fellow captives. After the Battle of Mobile Bay on August 5, 1864, for example, Surgeon Conrad and Assistant Surgeons Bowles and Booth helped treat the wounded Flag Officer Franklin Buchanan at the USN's hospital at Pensacola. Bowles and Booth were released in early September, and Conrad appears to have been released in late October of that year; a Southern newspaper reported that the prisoners had been "treated with courtesy and humanity." Assistant Surgeon Gibbes, captured on June 17, 1863, remained in captivity to treat his wounded comrades from the CSS *Atlanta*, was sent to Fort Warren, and was finally released on December 7, 1863. Surgeon Greenhow and contract surgeon Jones were paroled and released within two days of their capture near Roanoke Island in February 1862 because, according to Flag Officer L.M. Goldsborough, USN, "we could not conveniently dispose of them otherwise." On the other hand, Assistant Surgeon Emory, captured on October 7, 1864, was not released from Fort Warren until February 1, 1865, and his CSS *Florida* shipmate, Passed Assistant Surgeon Charlton, was confined in the same prison until June 30, 1865.[33]

It is difficult to generalize about the harshness of confinement

8. Surgeons Afloat

for CSN surgeons or about whether their treatment differed substantially from that of other imprisoned officers. Several surgeons were sent to Fort Warren, which was known during the first half of the war for its relatively kind treatment of inmates; conditions there became harsher later in the war after a change in prison commandants. Assistant Surgeon Bowles, of CSS *Tennessee*, remembered his USN captors kindly: "Indeed, they accorded us generous treatment as foemen worthy of their steel and soon the Blue and the Gray were fraternizing in the most friendly manner. The transition from hard-tack and Confederate coffee to three courses at a meal, supplemented with wine, on the elegant quarter of the [USS] Hartford and the [USS] Richmond, was something phenomenal." Later in the war, Bowles fell into the hands of Union troops under the command of Major General Philip Sheridan. Those soldiers, recalled Bowles, "marched me and starved me until I became so thin and shadowy, I escaped at night unobserved through the guards."[34]

* * *

Service aboard a war vessel entailed many routine tasks but also included the possibility of encounters with the enemy and the hazards of injury or capture. High among the responsibilities of naval surgeons were taking steps to promote the overall health of the crews and ensuring that their vessels were supplied and personnel trained for an efficient medical response in battle.

– 9 –

Medical Purveying

The CSN devoted relatively few men to the endeavor of obtaining and issuing drugs and other medical supplies—a task known, in the military, as medical purveying—yet those items were vital for the provision of care for sick or injured sailors. Appreciating the difficulty of medical purveying for the CSN requires an understanding of the market for medical goods before and during the Civil War.

Medicines in the Prewar Market

Medicinal articles in well-stocked pharmacies during the mid–1800s can be classified into three broad categories. The first consisted of raw materials, such as plant parts—seeds, bark, and roots, for example—and minerals. Such substances could be incorporated directly into medicines given to patients. The second category consisted of products manufactured from raw materials by pharmacists of ordinary skill, if they were so inclined. Such products could include tinctures or extracts or, in the case of nonvegetable raw materials, chemicals such as acids or chloroform. Items in this category were somewhat standardized in concentration and could be given directly to patients or included in compounded prescriptions. The third category consisted of items that ordinary pharmacists could not produce because they lacked the necessary knowledge, equipment, or time. A prime example is quinine, which was manufactured by a sophisticated process from the bark of South American cinchona trees. Only two American firms, both based in Philadelphia, manufactured quinine during the Civil War, and large quantities were made in England, France, and Germany.[1]

9. Medical Purveying

Although some raw medicinal materials were available in North America, many had to be imported. Imports also included manufactured items that were relatively simple—tinctures, extracts, and the like—and those that required complex processing, such as quinine. Almost all importation of medicinal articles occurred at Northern ports, particularly New York City, followed by Boston, Philadelphia, and Baltimore. Pharmacists and drug wholesalers from all parts of the United States, including the South, obtained their goods through Northern importers or wholesalers based near the large ports. Physicians who dispensed their own medicines often bought from local wholesalers whose goods had originally arrived through Northern ports. Large American drug manufacturers were located almost exclusively in the North.[2]

Prewar business between Northern suppliers and Southern customers was robust until secession and armed conflict seemed likely. At that point, some Northern suppliers started to decline Southern orders because they feared they would not receive payment. Similarly, some Southern customers stopped ordering from the North for fear that would not be able to pay or that the goods would not be delivered. Adding to concerns was a tariff imposed by the Confederate government on goods arriving from the North staring in March 1861. Some Southern wholesalers sought to build up their stock by placing large orders with Northern suppliers before the tariff took effect.[3]

Once hostilities began in April 1861, President Lincoln imposed a blockade of the ports of seven seceding state and then of two additional states. Lincoln also prohibited commercial dealings, unless exceptions were granted, between the Northern and seceding states. Among the items considered contraband by U.S. officials were medicines and surgical instruments, goods that originated in the North or in Europe.[4]

Purchasers and users of medicines had to be wary of impure, adulterated, or poor-quality goods, which were common in the marketplace. Drug adulteration, typically done by diluting raw materials with cheaper substances, was performed both overseas and by middlemen domestically. Purchasers, unprotected by effective regulation of the market, could partially guard against poor-quality drugs by dealing with reputable wholesalers and learning how to critically examine goods offered for sale.[5]

Ensuring consistent and acceptable drug quality was an impetus for the USN's Bureau of Medicine and Surgery to establish, in the early 1850s, the naval laboratory at the Brooklyn Naval Hospital. Before long, that facility was not only analyzing pharmaceutical ingredients and products contemplated for purchase by the navy, but also manufacturing high-quality medicines for the USN's use. By 1855, most medical supplies, including drugs and surgical instruments, issued to vessels and stations emanated from the laboratory. Thus, at the outset of the Civil War, USN medical officers had a table—appearing in the booklet *Instructions for the Government of the Medical Officers of the Navy of the United States*, the last prewar edition of which appears to have been published in 1857—showing the maximum amounts of medicines and other items that were allowed for vessels of various sizes. Requisitions for items on the list were sent directly to the Naval Laboratory, where personnel filled the orders by drawing from the available stock or by purchasing the needed articles on the open market. Whether a surgeon needed an ounce of quinine, a scalpel, a funnel, a bed pan, a pillow case, a candlestick, or a bottle of ink, he could request it from the Brooklyn laboratory.[6]

The South's Situation

With the outbreak of the war came a marked reduction of goods arriving from the North and a gradually more efficient blockade of Southern ports. Even in the case of items that did not have to be imported, the South was hampered by lacking a strong industrial base and enough experts to quickly start manufacturing medicines, surgical instruments, and other medical items. Thus, the OMS could not hope to immediately emulate the central procurement, examination, and distribution of medical supplies as practiced by the Brooklyn naval laboratory, whose personnel had practically unlimited buying opportunities in New York City.

9. Medical Purveying

For the OMS, the available options were to purchase on the open market—primarily through buying from Southern drug wholesalers or bidding at auction for goods delivered by blockade-runners—and buying foreign goods, through agents, before they arrived in the South. Such purchases would ideally be made by persons able to recognize high-quality goods. Although Southern wholesalers may have had ample inventories before war broke out, they had to replenish their stock by purchasing supplies arriving through the blockade, primarily at Wilmington and Charleston. Some medical supplies were smuggled from the North or captured by Confederate forces, but the contribution of such goods to the CSN's stock is not known.

European goods were typically shipped on large vessels to the neutral ports of Nassau (on New Providence in the Bahamas) and Bermuda—and less frequently to Havana—where cargoes were exchanged for cotton destined for Europe. The European goods were transferred to relatively small, swift ships that could more easily slip by the USN's blockading fleet and into a Southern port, where cargoes were offloaded and cotton was taken on for delivery to Nassau or Bermuda. The CSN, through agents, could buy goods not only in Europe but also at Nassau or Bermuda, since much of the cargo arriving the latter points had not been reserved for the Confederate government and was intended for sale to whomever would offer the best price, wherever that might be.[7]

Goods that arrived at Southern ports and subsequently offered for sale were often of dubious quality. As one observer described soon after the war:

> The wants of the Southern section of our country during the war had chiefly been supplied by foreign and domestic adventurers, through the means of blockade runners; and the risk of this species of illegitimate trade, coupled with the cupidity of those engaged in this contraband traffic, induced the parties concerned in it to export from abroad, and to import to the South very many deteriorated and factitious articles of medicine, because of their price, that in case of seizure their losses might not be so great. The consequence was, the South was but scantily supplied with medicines, and very many of those they had were of inferior character, and such as would not have been used in times of peace.[8]

The Confederate Navy Medical Corps

The OMS created its own version of the USN booklet and called it *Instructions for the Guidance of the Medical Officers of the Navy of the Confederate States*, with an 1862 issue date. Although the USN and CSN booklets resembled each other, the table of allowances in the CSN version differed somewhat from its USN counterpart. Whereas the USN's table indicated allowances for vessels of different size, the CSN version had allowances for one year for 100 men, a format used by the U.S. Army in its standard supply table for general and post hospitals. In addition, in the selection of drugs—and in how those drugs were named—the CSN list resembled the 1861 U.S. Army standard supply table more than the table in the 1857 USN booklet. The OMS, however, seemed fairly liberal in approving the purchase of items that were absent from its official list of allowances. That list, for example, omitted ether, but the widely used anesthetic was purchased by the CSN.[9]

The CSN's booklet instructed medical officers to submit requisitions quarterly to the OMS. Although the procedure implied an intent to fulfill requisitions centrally, medical officers were allowed to purchase supplies locally and account for them when completing their quarterly requisitions. Some of the earliest purchases—surgical instruments bought in or shipped to Montgomery (before the government's move to Richmond)—suggest that a single distribution hub at the capital was intended.[10]

Available records, however, indicate that a large portion of supplies, particularly in the first several months of the war, were obtained by medical officers locally rather than received by requisition from Montgomery or Richmond. Medicines and other supplies were purchased by Surgeon Francis L. Galt at New Orleans for CSS *Sumter* in June 1861, Assistant Surgeon Robert R. Gibbes at Savannah for CSS *Lady Davis* in June 1861, and Assistant Surgeon Frederic Van Bibber at Fredericksburg for CSS *Rappahannock* in August 1861. Confederate cruisers were sometime replenished with medical supplies overseas. While CSS *Florida* was docked at Brest, France, for example, its medical officers obtained medicines from a Brest pharmacy and medical textbooks from Paris. In the South, supplies were also bought locally for various naval stations and squadrons. At times, commanders of

9. Medical Purveying

vessels approved the purchase of medical supplies—selected by a surgeon's steward or hospital steward, when no medical officer was present—as happened for CSS *Huntress* at Savannah in December 1861 and CSS *Chattahoochee* at Columbus, Georgia, in March 1864.[11]

CSN surgeons wishing to purchase supplies locally had to compete with other potential buyers, who might include speculators, and even with Confederate army medical purveyors. It seems likely that army and naval buyers agreed not to compete for supplies in the same markets, although documentation of such cooperation has not been found. At times, naval medical buyers turned to the army for assistance. For example, Assistant Surgeon for the War Edwin G. Booth, CSN, serving with a detachment of Confederate marines at Drewry's Bluff, Virginia, requested and received an ambulance from the army medical department. Army medical officers who handled CSN requests for medical supplies included Surgeons Howard Smith, medical purveyor at Jackson, Mississippi, or Little Rock, Arkansas, in August 1862; Richard Potts, medical purveyor at Jackson, in September 1862; Nathaniel S. Crowell, medical director at Jackson, in December 1862; and Thomas Lining, medical purveyor at Charleston in 1862 and 1863.[12]

By early 1862, substantial amounts of medical supplies were being issued from Richmond, where the OMS purchased them primarily from Richmond wholesaler Purcell, Ladd and Company. In March 1862, OMS chief Spotswood called that firm the bureau's principal furnisher and reported to Secretary Mallory that the wholesaler could no longer fill orders because its last clerks and packers had been drafted into the Virginia Militia. Unless those employees could be exempted, said Spotswood, "our Naval vessels and Stations cannot be sufficiently supplied with medicines & Hospital Stores." The matter was referred to President Davis, who ordered that the employees be exempted from conscription.[13]

The CSN's Medical Purveying Department

By September 1862, the OMS was purchasing medicines and other supplies in Richmond for what it called the "medical purveyor's department," and by December 1862, Assistant Surgeon Charles M. Morfit was signing himself as "in charge" of the department, which was also called a store or storeroom. Historian John Coski places the navy's purveying department near the corner of 12th and Clay Streets in Richmond, although there is some indication that it shared the same building as the CSN Naval Hospital on 13th (or Governor) Street, between Franklin and Main Streets. Activities in the purveying department included buying and packing supplies for shipment. One probable example of the purveying department buying outside of Richmond was the forwarding from Charleston to Richmond of a shipment of medicines in November 1862 by Surgeon William F. Patton, surgeon of station at Charleston. OMS chief Spotswood reported in November 1863 that a large portion of supplies were purchased on the open market in Richmond and elsewhere. It has not been determined to what extent Spotswood dispatched agents to various spots in the South to purchase supplies or directed medical officers stationed at those places to buy goods and ship them to Richmond. In any event, Spotswood cited the blockade as contributing to the "enormous cost" of the OMS's purchases.[14]

One drawback of having Richmond as the sole hub for the distribution of medical supplies was that blockade-running vessels did not arrive there. Unlike New York City, where goods of all descriptions arrived and could be purchased for the USN's Brooklyn laboratory, the OMS, for much of the war, had to rely on goods arriving primarily at Wilmington and Charleston, compete against other buyers, and settle for what it could get. Purchases would then have to be shipped on inefficient railroads to Richmond to fill requisitions from various points in the Confederacy, including Wilmington and Charleston. It seems odd that the OMS did not establish regional purveying depots at those two cities to save freight expenses and hasten deliveries.

Spotswood suggested in November 1863 that a competent apothecary be sent to Europe to buy medical supplies and ship them to Bermuda. Although contractors had been hired to do the same, Spotswood considered them "not competent to make the proper selection" and believed them to be concerned with "important and more lucrative interests ... which may lead to a neglect of this

9. Medical Purveying

department." At that time, Spotswood worried that an increasingly efficient Federal navy might prevent blockade-runners from entering the port of Wilmington and severely compromise his European supply line.[15]

Assistant Surgeon Morfit's term in charge of the medical purveying department lasted until early February 1863, when he was transferred to the Charleston Squadron to serve on CSS *Stono*. Purchases in Richmond in February through May 1863 for items suitable for outfitting and stocking an apothecary were made by Passed Assistant Surgeon James W. Herty. By May 1863, Spotswood hired civilian druggist Robert Lecky, who was paid for "apothecary & dispensing duties." Among the nondrug items purchased by Lecky for the department were "laboratory instruments and utensils." By the next month, Lecky was signing himself as apothecary in charge of the medical purveying department.[16]

Lecky appears to have been responsible for selecting and purchasing supplies in Richmond and directing their packing and delivery to various points in the South. He was assisted by at least two other druggists, one of whom was George Dowden; the other has not been identified. OMS chief Spotswood described the apothecaries' duties as "manufacturing, receiving, packing, and issuing medicines." Dowden appears to have been regularly assigned to accompany supplies to various naval stations. In fall 1863, for example, his delivery route took him to Wilmington, Charleston, Savannah, and St. Marks, Florida. During that trip, he arranged for transport of supplies from Quitman, Georgia, to Monticello, Florida. Later that year, he traveled to Wilmington and Mobile. Spotswood reported having to hire additional messengers frequently "to comply with requisitions from small places between this city [Richmond] and Mobile." Spotswood appealed to Secretary Mallory to protect his druggists from active army duty and being replaced by disabled soldiers: "Crippled soldiers and men exempted by reason of ill health, and not experts, would not answer the purposes of the purveyor's department, since they would be incompetent to the discharge of the duties required in the transportation and selection of proper and pure medicines ordered to be purchased from time to time."[17]

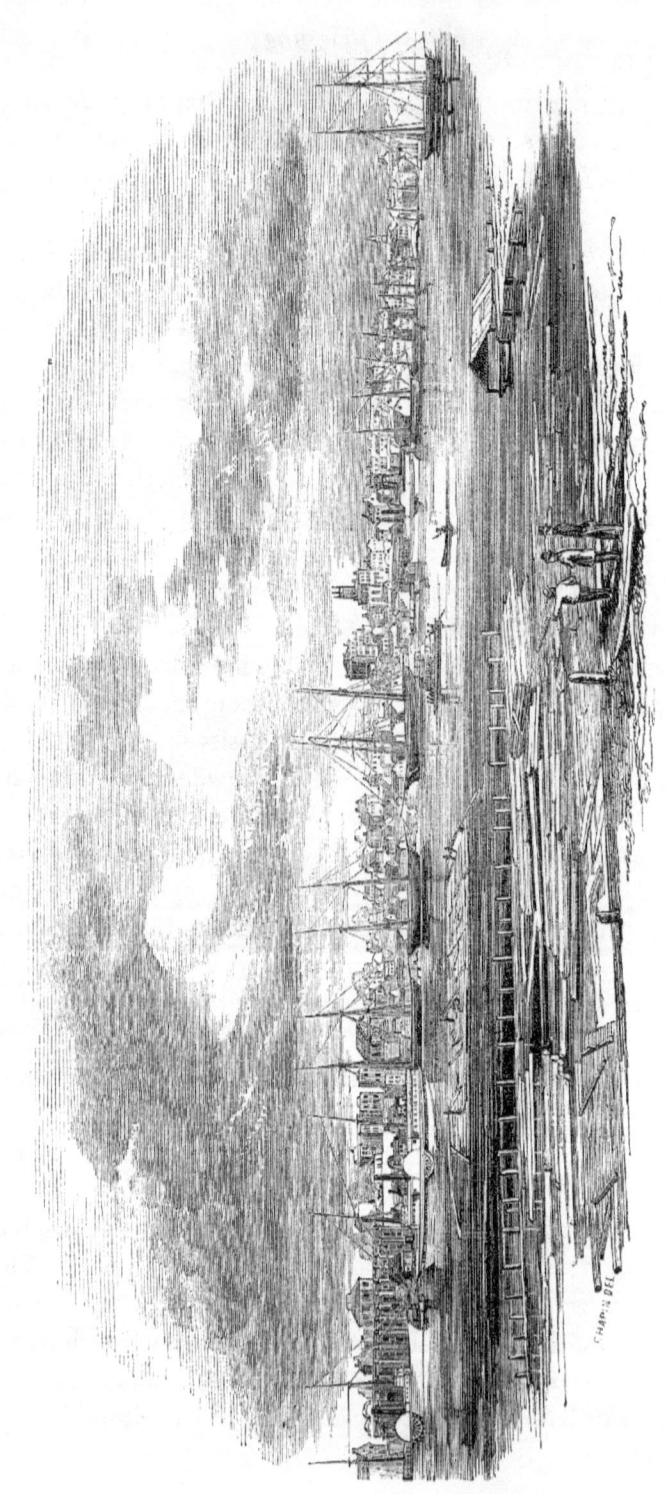

Wilmington, North Carolina: a key destination for blockade-runners; site of an 1862 epidemic of yellow fever; and home to a Confederate naval station, squadron, and hospital (*Gleason's Pictorial Drawing-Room Companion*, July 16, 1853).

9. Medical Purveying

Dowden's deliveries to the naval station at St. Marks, near Tallahassee, were not sufficient to serve the needs of that facility. Thus, in May 1863, Assistant Surgeon John DeBree, Jr., was ordered by the commander of CSS *Spray*, Lieutenant Charles W. Hays, to proceed to Quincy, Florida, to obtain medical supplies for the vessel from the army medical purveyor there (probably Surgeon John E.A. Davidson). About a year later, Assistant Surgeon James V. Cook, stationed at St. Marks, was ordered by the Office of Orders and Detail to proceed to Richmond to take charge of medicines for the St. Marks naval station. If the supplies had been scrutinized by medical officers at Quincy and Richmond, it would seem that a surgeon's steward or civilian agent could have handled such missions.[18]

In November 1863 and November 1864, Spotswood reported that the purveying department had successfully furnished all vessels and stations with sufficient supplies. Despite that claim, numerous local purchases were still being made for individual vessels and naval stations. In addition, the commander of at least one commerce raider, *Tallahassee*, was ordered in July 1864 to preserve "the medicine chests of captured and destroyed vessels, and all drugs and medicines," an action that would have been unnecessary if adequate supplies were readily available to the CSN. Contributing to the purveying department's reported success was Lecky's ability to manufacture certain medicines at lower-than-market costs. Spotswood's 1863 report listed 18 such medicines. Most were identical or similar to items on the official list of allowances of medical supplies. Lecky was able to make tincture of opium, for example, for $6.00 a pound, compared with the market price of $9.00, but his expense in producing syrup of squills ($3.50 per pound) exceeded the market price ($1.85). Spotswood did not report Lecky's total production or the amount of money saved by his efforts. It is not known whether the OMS attempted to establish multiple drug-manufacturing laboratories, as the Confederate army did, to supplement Lecky's endeavors in Richmond.[19]

Additional evidence that Spotswood's purveying department was having difficulties obtaining adequate supplies of medicines comes from the examination of some of the CSN's purchases. The surgeon general of the Confederate army, Samuel Preston Moore, had responded to drug shortages by encouraging the use of medicines made from native plants. Many such medicines were known to physicians but were not considered first-line therapies. They might, however, still prove useful, and part of Moore's effort was the distribution of three publications meant to educate medical officers—and possibly the public—about the usefulness of indigenous resources. These included a short pamphlet issued in 1862, a standard supply table of indigenous remedies issued in 1863, and an 1863 book titled *Resources of the Southern Fields and Forests*, by Confederate army surgeon Francis Peyre Porcher.[20]

The CSN purveying department, under Assistant Surgeon Morfit, purchased some tincture of lobelia (*Lobelia inflata*, Indian tobacco) in November 1862. After Robert Lecky was hired in May 1863, purchases included a copy of Porcher's book, spigelia (*Spigelia marilandica*, pink root) root, and boneset (*Eupatorium perfoliatum*). Neither lobelia, spigelia, nor boneset were in the CSN's standard supply table, but all were included in the three publications issued at Surgeon General Moore's direction. Whereas army medical purveyors encouraged citizens to collect and dry medicinal plants for sale to army medical laboratories, the CSN bought its lobelia and spigelia from wholesaler Purcell, Ladd and Company. in Richmond. At least some of the CSN's boneset (87 pounds) was obtained from one F.H. Robertson, but whether Robertson was a wholesaler has not been determined. Extract of boneset was among the formulations prepared by Lecky.[21]

OMS chief Spotswood reported in November 1864 that all naval hospitals had "been well provided for with clean and comfortable bedding, blankets, furniture, crockery, etc." by buying the items at auction at "200 per cent less"—perhaps meaning a third—of what Richmond wholesalers were charging. At that time, Spotswood also mentioned that "by the employment of an upholsterer in the purveyor's department to remodel and renovate beds, much expense has been saved."[22]

It has not been determined whether the OMS contracted with local artisans to make surgical instruments and other nondrug medical supplies. Among the items made by local manufacturers for the Confederate army medical department were surgical instruments, bedding, hospital clothing, and cots. The quality of the resultant surgical instruments was generally poor. The CSN's Mobile Squadron called on L. Koch to repair surgical instruments in 1862 and 1864 for CSS *Baltic* and in 1864 for CSS *Selma*, and the Savannah Squadron had E.L. Harley clean and repair a case of instruments in 1864, but records do not indicate where the articles were made or why they required repair.[23]

The CSN did call on patriotic ladies to make roller bandages—"to be one, two, three, and four inches wide, and of any length"—and to scrape lint for use in dressings. In that case, contributions were to be sent to Assistant Surgeon William Mason Turner at Charleston's naval rendezvous.[24]

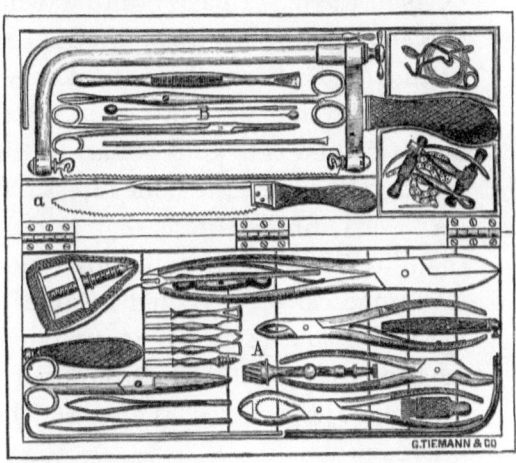

Surgical set of a type needed by CSN surgeons. High-quality instruments were made in Europe or the Northern states and entered the South via blockade-running or smuggling across enemy lines. This set, from the New York firm of George Tiemann and Company, featured a removable tray (top), amputation saws, knives, and a tourniquet (*The American Armamentarium Chirurgicum* [New York: George Tiemann, 1889]).

The Blockade's Tightening Grip

What CSN medical officers paid for quinine gives some indication of rising prices in the South. In May 1861, quinine was purchased in New Orleans for $3 an ounce (in Confederate dollars), and by June 1863, the drug was bought for $25 an ounce in Savannah and

Richmond. The July 1863 loss of Vicksburg, which effectively relinquished Confederate control of the Mississippi River, was followed by a rise in the per-ounce price to $40 at Mobile in September 1863 and to $125 at Marion Court House, South Carolina, in November 1864. In Shreveport, which was cut off from the blockade-running ports of the East Coast, quinine (when it could be obtained at all) was selling for $325–$350 an ounce in summer 1864. The rise in price from $3 (New Orleans, May 9, 1861) to $125 (Marion Court House, November 8, 1864) represents a 41.7-fold increase, whereas the price of a U.S. gold dollar, in Confederate currency in Richmond, rose during the same interval from $1.12 to $28.00, a 25-fold increase. Quinine's increase in price, which occurred more quickly than the Confederate dollar lost value, reflected the difficulty that CSN medical officers had in obtaining it. Although a growing need for medical services necessitated higher Congressional appropriations for the OMS throughout the war, the increases were unlikely to have allowed the bureau's buying power to keep pace with inflation.[25]

By November 1, 1864, Spotswood considered the USN to have essentially closed the Confederacy's East Coast ports to blockade-runners, so he ordered medical officers at the various stations to buy supplies locally. (The last steam-powered blockade-runner arrived at Wilmington around December 28, 1864.) Surgeon William E. Wysham at Mobile identified himself as representing the medical purveying department when buying from local dealers in 1864. In May 1864, Wysham placed an order forwarded by Paymaster Thomas R. Ware to Charles J. Helm, Confederate agent in Havana. That or a similar order appears to have been filled, at least in part, by a shipment on the British steamer *Denbigh*, which made frequent trips between Havana and Mobile. Surgeon William Meade Page, serving at Shreveport, was ordered in February 1864 to buy medical supplies in Houston, where goods that had been shipped from Havana to Galveston might be available.[26]

9. Medical Purveying

Medicinal Alcohol

Having adequate supplies of alcohol was of particular concern to the CSN and involved both the Office of Provisions and Clothing and the OMS. Sailors were entitled, as part of their daily ration, to a gill (four ounces) of spirits (typically whiskey) or a half pint of wine; those forgoing the spirit ration received a daily commutation of four cents, which represented the item's cost. The spirit ration was provided by the Office of Provisions and Clothing. Medicinal alcohol, on the other hand, differed from the spirit ration in that it was used to treat patients and not supplied routinely to healthy sailors. Surgeons considered alcohol a medical necessity, and it appeared on the OMS's table of allowances in the form of an 85 percent alcohol solution (simply called *alcohol* by the United States Pharmacopoeia and not meant for internal use unless diluted), brandy, wine, and ale or porter. The OMS was responsible for purchasing medicinal alcohol.[27]

Early in the war, the Office of Provisions and Clothing could buy barreled whiskey, for the spirit ration, for 31–50 cents a gallon. There being 32 daily rations per gallon, the commutation of four cents, represented more than the spirit's cost. By November 1863, Paymaster John DeBree, Sr., of the Office of Provisions and Clothing, reported that ordinary grades of whiskey cost $50–$75 per gallon, an expenditure that did not warrant its issue. Contracts with distillers had been unsuccessful, and if the navy wanted to continue the spirit ration, DeBree recommended establishing government distilleries and raising the commutation to 10 or even 20 cents a day, which would be well short of the current cost of the spirit ration of about $2. Erecting distilleries, however, would violate states laws that prohibited the production of alcohol; various governors believed that grain should instead feed their citizens or soldiers. By order of Secretary Mallory, the spirit ration was suspended on November 23, 1863, and evidently never reinstated.[28]

Medical officers purchased medicinal alcohol before and after suspension of the spirit ration. Whiskey, although not included in the table of allowances, could be used in place of the other listed alcoholic beverages and was usually, but not always, less expensive.

The Confederate Navy Medical Corps

At Savannah, medical officers bought brandy for $2.75 per bottle in August 1862 and for $25 per bottle in January 1864. In July 1864, Assistant Surgeon Joel G. King paid $80 for a half gallon of whiskey for CSS *Neuse*.[29]

To help supply the OMS and allow reinstatement of the spirit ration, naval agent William F. Howell of the Office of Provisions and Clothing arranged for the building of a distillery near Augusta, Georgia. Construction of another began somewhere in South Carolina. Secretary Mallory reported that the governor of South Carolina, Milledge L. Bonham, ordered that work on the distillery in his state be stopped. Mallory referred the matter to the Confederate attorney general, George Davis, who opined that the governor's order had no legal standing. In response to the Confederate army encountering similar opposition to contracting with distillers or establishing its own distilleries, the Confederate Congress enacted a law in June 1864 authorizing such activity on the part of the army surgeon general and commissary general. The law did not mention the CSN, and it is unclear how many distilleries the navy established or how effective they were in providing affordable whiskey.[30]

* * *

The OMS devoted personnel to the task of purchasing, and in some cases, manufacturing medical necessities. Despite reassurances by OMS chief Spotswood that naval stations and vessels were adequately supplied with those items, evidence suggests that the blockade and rising prices resulted in naval surgeons not always having the drugs, instruments, and other supplies that they needed.

– 10 –

Hospitals

The CSN established multiple shore-based hospitals and a small but unknown number of floating hospitals. They were intended to care for personnel whose illnesses or injuries were such that they were unlikely to recover in their own quarters or on a nonhospital vessel. When CSN hospitals were not conveniently nearby, the unusual practice was to transfer patients to army hospitals or have them visited by civilian physicians in civilian-operated hospitals or in some convenient structure near a naval station.

One example of a civilian-run hospital was the Charity Hospital in New Orleans, a state institution that admitted sailors from vessels of the Mississippi River Squadron and from the hospital ship *St. Philip* during at least the latter part of 1861. Another example was the Soldier's Home in Columbus, Georgia—also called the Ladies Hospital because of its establishment by the Ladies Soldier's Friend Society. Opened in May 1862, the Soldier's Home received sick or injured crewmembers from CSS *Chattahoochee* at least three times, the patients being escorted there by the vessel's assistant surgeon, Marcellus Ford. One of those occurrences was after *Chattahoochee*'s boiler exploded in May 1863. According to one officer, the patients "received all the attention that could possibly have been bestowed…. The four worst cases were placed together in the room upstairs…. It was with the utmost difficulty that I could remain in the room sufficiently long to ascertain what was required and to see what service I could render, the atmosphere [odor] was so unpleasant, yet the ladies did not seem to notice it and remained at their post till the last." At least two civilian physicians, A.C. Wingfield and E.F. Colzey, attended patients at Soldier's Home and were contract surgeons for the army, but it is unclear whether the army had any formal association with Soldier's Home at the time.[1]

In several instances, the CSN rented buildings as hospitals and staffed them with naval and civilian personnel. Available records do not show that the CSN built its own hospitals, although it certainly modified rented structures to better serve as hospitals. Naval shore facilities, such as shipyards, typically had a medical officer and steward on duty. Such locales probably included an infirmary where sick or injured personnel could seek care; the most serious cases could be sent to a naval or civilian hospital or prompt a call to a local physician to render care or provide advice.

Pensacola

The CSN's first hospital was obtained when Florida and Alabama troops seized the Federal naval facilities at the Pensacola Navy Yard in January 1861. (The yard was actually contiguous with the town of Warrington and several miles southwest of the city of Pensacola. Although *Pensacola* seems to have been part of the official name of the yard and hospital, the facilities were often described more accurately as being at Warrington.) The Pensacola Naval Hospital, often mistakenly called the Marine Hospital, was not in the yard proper but rather about three quarters of a mile west of it; about a half mile to the west of the hospital was Fort Barrancas. William Whelan, chief of the USN's Bureau of Medicine and Surgery, described the hospital as "erected on a bluff overlooking the [Pensacola] Bay and Gulf of Mexico, the labor of many years, and much money." USN medical officers serving at the naval hospital in January 1861 were Surgeon Spotswood, who resigned from the USN a few days after the yard was seized, and Passed Assistant Surgeon William F. Carrington, who resigned from the USN in March 1861. During January, direction of the hospital appears to have assigned to Dr. William D. Lyles from Mississippi, who signed himself variously as "Surgeon General," "Surgeon in Charge," and "Surgeon in Chief."[2]

In February 1861, hospital steward F.R. Hacklander reported a single patient being in the hospital, whose staff also included a matron, a nurse, a cook, and three watchmen. The navy yard proper

10. Hospitals

appears to have had its own dispensary and medical storeroom, the keys to which were surrendered by Passed Assistant Surgeon William S. Bishop, USN, in January 1861. After the Confederate government assumed control of the yard in March 1861, Secretary Mallory estimated that the yard would require, among other officers, one surgeon and one surgeon's steward, while the hospital would require one surgeon, one assistant surgeon, one surgeon's steward, one matron, three nurses, two cooks, three washers, one carter, one messenger, and three watchmen. CSN medical officers present at Warrington (or at least on the payroll there) during 1861 and 1862 included Spotswood, who was paid through May 8, 1861, Carrington, who was paid through June 1861, and Assistant Surgeon Joseph D. Grafton, Jr., who was paid from July 1861 (at the latest) through January 1862.[3]

Federal advances during the first quarter of 1862 prompted Confederate commanders to concentrate their resources, which necessitated the abandonment of the Pensacola Navy Yard and the destruction of anything there that might be useful to the Union military. Having completed the removal of heavy guns, ammunition, troops, and the wounded, Acting Brigadier General Thomas M. Jones, commanding at Warrington, ordered the destruction of naval property at and surrounding the yard, including the naval hospital. Fires were ignited shortly before midnight on May 9, 1862, and by daybreak, the yard and hospital were in ashes, and the area was too hot to enter. In 1863, Surgeon William Whelan, chief of the USN's Bureau of Medicine and Surgery, reported that "the destruction of the [hospital] building and its contents is believed to have been complete." Details about the operation of the Pensacola Naval Hospital while under Confederate control have not been found.[4]

After the USN repossessed the yard, it constructed a temporary hospital building, apparently within the yard, in 1863 and enlarged it during the war. Among the patients treated there were CSN and USN crewmembers of vessels engaged in the Battle of Mobile Bay in August 1864. The most prominent of those patients was Flag Officer Franklin Buchanan, CSN, who had sustained a serious leg injury. The Confederate wounded from the battle were accompanied by CSN medical officers Fleet Surgeon Daniel B. Conrad and Assistant

Surgeons Edwin G. Booth and Richard C. Bowles. Conrad described the hospital as "large" and "ample." In 1875, the USN constructed another hospital outside of the yard, atop the ruins of the original hospital.[5]

Norfolk

In some ways, the history of the CSN's hospital at Norfolk, Virginia, paralleled that of its hospital at Pensacola. On April 17, 1861, the Virginia State Convention adopted an ordinance of secession. Fearing a takeover of the yard by Virginia state troops, and with instructions not to leave valuable resources to insurrectionists, Commodore C.S. McCauley, USN, commandant of the yard, ordered the destruction of property there and abandonment of the yard on April 20. Among the structures left unharmed was the naval hospital. A Virginia official described the facility: "The naval hospital near Portsmouth is located at the most beautiful and healthy point in the harbor. It is built of free stone and granite, and is capable of accommodating 600 patients. It is provided with every convenience and appliance needed for the objects for which it was designed. All the necessary dependencies for a first-class hospital, such as surgeon's dwellings, keeper's house, cemetery, stables, etc., are provided; and the grounds are covered with a growth of shade trees." The hospital—which was across the Elizabeth River from Norfolk—was separated by the town of Portsmouth from the yard, which was contiguous with the town of Gosport; the hospital and yard were about a mile and a half apart. The names of Norfolk, Portsmouth, and Gosport were all used when referring to the hospital The value of medical stores lost at Norfolk by the USN was about $400 on the receiving ship *Pennsylvania*, $500 at the navy yard, and $6,400 at the hospital.[6]

USN medical officers serving or residing nearby in early 1861 included Surgeons Lewis W. Minor, Randolph F. Mason, and William B. Sinclair and Passed Assistant Surgeons William E. Wysham and Charles H. Williamson, all of whom tendered their resignations from the USN between April 17 and 25, 1861, and became medical

10. Hospitals

officers in the CSN. The Norfolk naval facilities were controlled by the Virginia navy until June 6, 1861, when they were transferred to the Confederate States. During that time, Surgeon Minor served there as a member of the Virginia navy. The grounds around the hospital, which had been built on the site of the old Fort Nelson, were fortified and again called Fort Nelson.[7]

Little is known about the operation of the hospital while under CSN control. By July 1, 1861, Surgeon Minor, now in the CSN, had been transferred to New Orleans, and by October 1861, Surgeon William F. Patton was signing vouchers for supplies needed at the navy yard. Surgeon George Blacknall served for an unknown duration at the hospital before dying of pneumonia on January 20, 1862. By that time, the facility was controlled by the army and was called the General Hospital at Norfolk. On January 22, 1862, Surgeon James Cornick, CSN, was ordered to report to Major General Benjamin Huger, Commanding the Department of Norfolk, for duty at the general hospital.[8]

On March 11, 1862, Surgeon Francis Peyre Porcher of the Confederate army was assigned to take charge of the "General Hospital at Fort Nelson," a name possibly used to avoid calling the facility a naval hospital. Porcher called the hospital a "noble structure" and marveled that a barge was supplied for his use. One prominent patient treated at the facility was Flag Officer Franklin Buchanan, who had been aboard CSS *Virginia* during the Battle of Hampton Roads on March 8, 1862, and sustained a dangerous leg wound that necessitated a lengthy hospitalization; Lieutenant R.D. Minor, and probably other CSN personnel wounded in the battle, were treated at the hospital. Naval officers continued to call the facility the "Naval Hospital," and naval personnel continued to be treated there at least through March 1862.[9]

The approach of Union forces prompted the CSN to set fire to and evacuate the Norfolk Navy Yard on May 9, 1862. The hospital, again spared, was reoccupied by the USN around September 1, 1862. "Besides being stripped of its furniture and left in an exceedingly filthy condition," reported Surgeon William Whelan, USN, the hospital "sustained no great damage." The hospital building, in modified form, still stands as part of the Naval Medical Center Portsmouth.[10]

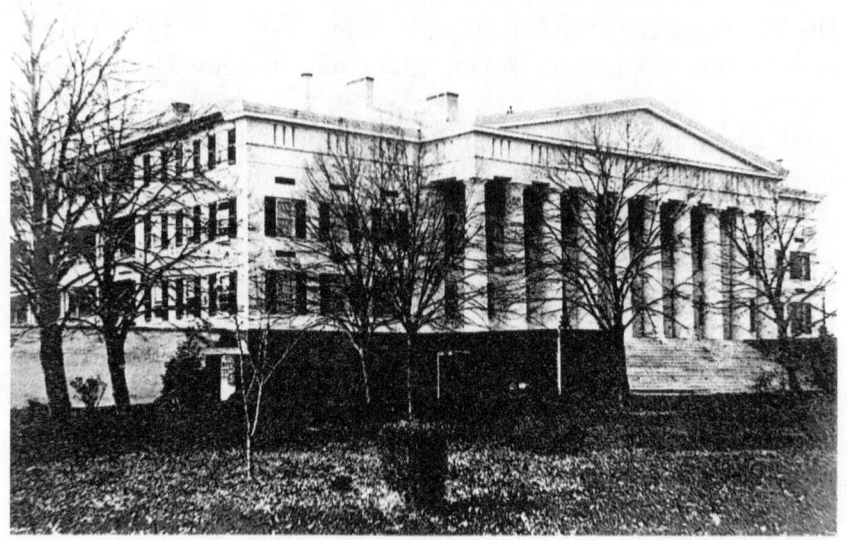

The Norfolk Naval Hospital in the mid–1870s. The facility was abandoned by the USN in April 1861, used by the Confederate navy and army, and left intact by Confederate forces when they left the area in May 1862 (Library of Congress, control no. va1555).

The histories of the Norfolk and Pensacola Navy Yards had numerous similarities. Both were originally USN facilities, were seized early in the war by Southern troops, were burned by withdrawing Confederate forces on May 9, 1862, were reoccupied by the USN, and had an associated hospital that treated Flag Officer Buchanan for a leg injury after a major naval battle.

Richmond

The Naval Hospital in Richmond was established about May 1, 1862, on 13th Street, between Main and Franklin Street. The structure, which evidently housed the hospital for the rest of the war, was rented from upholsterer William Ritter at $1,900 per year from May 1862 through April 1863. By mid–1863, the rent was $2,500 per year. In early 1865, Ritter petitioned the Confederate Congress for permission to increase the rent, but the request was tabled.[11]

10. Hospitals

OMS chief Spotswood and Surgeon Lewis W. Minor were initially in charge of hiring hospital personnel and having the building fitted out as a hospital. They advertised for a surgeon's steward, mechanics, a plumber, a bricklayer, African American nurses, and various servants. They hired contractors for carpentry and installation of water and gas fixtures, and they purchased cots, mattresses, and pillows. The hospital probably benefited by being on the same block as Purcell, Ladd and Company, the OMS's major supplier of medical goods in Richmond. Spotswood rented an ice house in Manchester, across the James River from Richmond, to provide for the hospital.[12]

By about July 1862, charge of the hospital appears to have been assigned to Surgeon James F. Harrison, who served in that position for most, if not all, of the remainder of the war. Harrison was assisted, at various times, by Passed Assistant Surgeon Marcellus P. Christian, Assistant Surgeon John DeBree, Jr., Assistant Surgeon Luther R. Dickinson, Assistant Surgeon John E. Duffel, Passed Assistant Surgeon Bennett W. Green, and Assistant Surgeon Joel G. King. On any particular day, some eight to 10 civilian employees were on duty. They typically included a steward, a ward master, a matron, a messenger, and a few nurses. Most or all of the nurses were men, and many were slaves hired from their owners. For example, in January 1863, Surgeon Harrison asked that the hospital payroll include four new nurses: Jesse Hampton, belonging to C.W. Hewlett; Flemming Dabney, belonging to Mrs. Wharton; Henry Bright, belonging to Robert Ould; and Griffin Peyton, belonging to Mr. Billups. The hospital's steward, Richard Hall, was sometimes paid to transport patients from the Richmond Navy Yard at Rocketts Landing, but by September 1863, the hospital had acquired an ambulance and had purchased a horse, bridle, and collar.[13]

At times, Richmond-area CSN patients were treated at an army hospital, such as Chimborazo Hospital No. 2, Howard's Grove Hospital, Jackson Hospital, or General Hospital No. 8, 9, 13, or 21. Some of these patients had known or suspected smallpox and were sent, evidently at the request of army medical authorities, to an army hospital that isolated and treated such cases. The army's General Hospital No. 21, for example, opened on November 18, 1862, to receive smallpox patients, and on December 9, 1862, Surgeon Harrison at the Richmond Naval Hospital transferred three such patients to that facility in conformity to a communication from the army medical director in Richmond. On the same day, Assistant Surgeon James E. Lindsay, CSN, serving at the batteries at Drewry's Bluff, requested that an unknown hospital (probably General Hospital No. 21) receive a patient with smallpox.[14]

In mid–1862, the Richmond Naval Hospital admitted army patients, some or all of whom had been wounded during recent combat near the city, possibly at the Seven Days' Battles. Although Richmond's army hospitals were estimated to have a capacity of 5,000–6,000 patients, they were overwhelmed with casualties resulting from the Union's Peninsular Campaign, and Confederate army medical authorities no doubt sought the CSN's assistance. Other instances of treating army patients in naval hospitals were probably uncommon.[15]

During the first three quarters of 1863, the Richmond Naval Hospital admitted 177 patients and discharged 159. During the next year, ending on October 1, 1864, the hospital admitted 842 patients and discharged 645; more than half of the year's admissions and discharges occurred during the third quarter of 1864, when malaria was particularly widespread in the James River Squadron. At one point in August 1864, 157 men from seven vessels were reported by the squadron's flag officer to be in the Richmond Naval Hospital. Although the capacity of the hospital is unknown, it seems unlikely that it normally had space for that many patients. If adequate room was not available, the hospital's medical officers probably had the option of transferring some patients to army hospitals. In late March 1865, Surgeon Harrison asked Levin Smith Joynes, the dean of MCV, whether that institution's infirmary was available for use as a naval hospital, but whether Joynes responded has not been determined.[16]

Mobile

The Naval Hospital at Mobile was evidently established no later than July 1, 1862, and occupied a building at the corner of St. Anthony

10. Hospitals

and Scott Streets in summer 1863. During 1864, rental payments of $150 per month for the hospital building were paid to the firm of Ross and Ketchum. Medical officers serving at the hospital at various times included Surgeon William E. Wysham (apparently in charge), Surgeon Algernon S. Garnett, and Assistant Surgeons Edwin G. Booth, William W. Graves, Jeptha V. Harris, and Robert C. Powell.[17]

On average, the hospital payroll included eight to 10 workers who were not officers. Some of those employees—laundresses, for example—were definitely civilians, but others had a job title, such as hospital steward or surgeon's steward, that might apply to a civilian or enlisted man. Starting in the third quarter of 1863, the hospital payroll included men assigned elsewhere: John J. Shepperd, the surgeon's steward of the Mobile Station; Emile Atsinger, the surgeon's steward of the Mobile Marine Barracks, and M.E. Wysham, clerk for the medical purveyor (probably related to hospital surgeon and medical purveyor William E. Wysham). Shepperd may not have been the first choice as surgeon's steward of Lewis W. Minor, surgeon of station at Mobile, for in October 1862, Surgeon Minor placed a notice in Richmond newspaper asking Robert H.F. McWilkie if he would accept the surgeon's stewardship at Mobile. McWilkie had evidently served in the USN with Minor, was at the USN's Norfolk Naval Hospital when it was abandoned in April 1861, and reenlisted in the USN in 1863.[18]

The Mobile Marine Barracks occupied the Matthews Press building and wharves on Commerce Street, below Church Street, and was rented for $4,000 per year from M. Waring Goodman and others. In mid–August 1864, after most of the marines at the barracks had participated in the Battle of Mobile Bay, Captain Ebenezer Farrand, commanding the Mobile Squadron, ordered Surgeon Minor to "take charge of all sick and wounded men who may be sent for treatment to the late Marine Barracks."[19]

Although the capacity of the Mobile Naval Hospital has not been determined, it had 41 patients on October 1, 1863. During the first three quarters of 1863, the hospital admitted 276 patients and discharged 232. From that date until October 1, 1864, the hospital admitted 372 patients and discharged 251.[20]

Assistant Surgeon Edwin G. Booth reported for duty at the

Mobile Naval Hospital on November 18, 1864, and was carried on the Mobile Station payroll for all of January 1865, the last month for which payroll records for that facility are available. Nevertheless, Booth was admitted to the army's Way Hospital in Meridian, Mississippi, on January 19 and March 2, 1865; no admitting diagnosis was recorded. It is not clear what these hospitalizations say about the operational status of the Mobile Naval Hospital in early 1865 or its ability to provide treatment for Booth specifically.[21]

Benton, Mississippi

A naval hospital associated with the Yazoo City (Mississippi) Navy Yard was established no earlier than October 1862, at Benton, Mississippi. At that time, Assistant Surgeon John Joseph Steinriede incurred expenses for the accommodation of sick men sent to Benton "before hospital arrangements were made." In late December 1862, Steinriede submitted a requisition for medical goods to Surgeon Nathaniel S. Crowell, an army medical director at Jackson, Mississippi. Crowell agreed to send a one-month supply. No other records of the Benton Naval Hospital have been found. The navy yard was evacuated in May 1863.[22]

Charleston

The CSN hospital in Charleston appears to have been established no later than April 1, 1863. In 1864, the hospital occupied a house—rented from F.J. Pelzer at $100 per month—at the corner of Spring and King Streets, but whether it was ever located elsewhere in the city is not clear. A Charleston newspaper indicated that the hospital was under the charge of Surgeon William F. Patton, who at the time was surgeon of station at Charleston. Among the other medical officers assigned to the hospital was Assistant Surgeon Robert R. Gibbes.[23]

The civilian staff, usually numbering eight or nine, was headed by steward John W. Evans, who was also the steward of the Charleston Marine Hospital on Franklin Street. That facility, formed to care

10. Hospitals

for seamen, evidently continued to do so while also admitting Confederate army patients. It was under the charge of the Charleston City Council and not part of the U.S. Treasury Department's system of marine hospitals. In September 1863, Evans was paid by the CSN for moving furniture, medicines, and other items from Franklin Street (probably the Marine Hospital) to Spring Street (probably the Naval Hospital). Among the civilian staff of the Naval hospital were four other persons named Evans: matron E.J. (possibly John Evans's wife, Emily), servant William (possibly Evans's son), cook Rose, and laundress Catey. Other civilian workers included a ward master, two or three nurses, and an apothecary.[24]

The hospital's capacity is unknown, but it had 23 patients on October 1, 1863. During the first three quarters of 1863, it admitted 149 patients and discharged 124. During the next year, it admitted 252 patients and discharged 154.[25]

On February 13, 1865, orders were given to evacuate Charleston, and Flag Officer Duncan N. Ingraham directed that the Charleston Naval Hospital be removed to a northern section of South Carolina, with the goal of settling at Chesterville (Chester). Passed Assistant Surgeon Frederic Garretson had been sent there by the OMS to prepare for the reception of personnel, patients, and all of the hospital fixtures, medical equipment, and supplies that could be transported. The whole, under charge of Passed Assistant Surgeon Robert R. Gibbes, suffered various delays on the railroads before arriving at Charlotte, North Carolina, on February 25. There, General P.G.T. Beauregard advised Gibbes to abandon any hope of reaching Chesterville but to instead set up the hospital at the base of the hill in Charlotte on which stood the North Carolina Military Institute. Gibbes ran the hospital there until April 14, when circumstances forced him to disband it. Gibbes bid farewell to his patients and advised them to make their way home as best they could.[26]

Savannah

Multiple buildings housed CSN patients in Savannah. The first, known as the City, Poor House, or Marine Hospital, admitted naval

The Confederate Navy Medical Corps

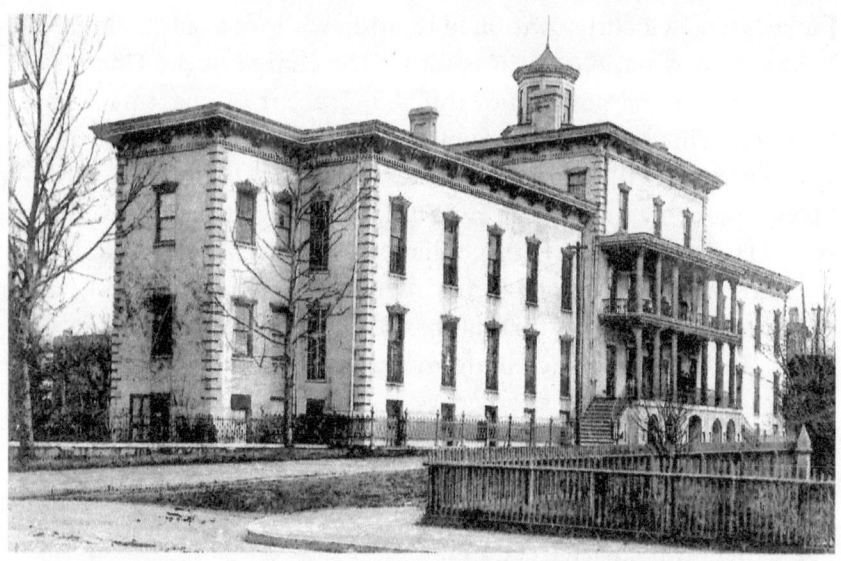

City Hospital (also called the Marine or Poor House Hospital) in Savannah. Early in the war, CSN patients were treated here by civilian physicians. The CSN later rented the building as a hospital (postcard photograph taken in the early 1900s, author's collection).

patients starting no later than late May 1861 and continued doing so through at least mid–July 1863. The structure, built in 1819, was bounded by Gaston and Huntingdon Streets on the north and south, respectively, and by Drayton and Abercorn Streets on the west and east, respectively; it was adjacent to an open space known as the South Commons. The building's original use as a hospital for sailors may have accounted for its being known as the Marine Hospital, although that name may also have arisen because the Marine Bank held its mortgage at one time; antebellum Savannah had no facility in the U.S. Treasury Department's system of marine hospitals. It appears that naval surgeons did not attend to patients at the City Hospital before mid–1863. Rather, the CSN paid the hospital for board and medicine and for care provided by the hospital's physicians.[27]

The CSN then took a year's lease for $5,000, starting in July 1863, on a hotel or inn known as the Gibbons House, at West Broad and Broughton Streets, and began outfitting it as a hospital in July and

10. Hospitals

August 1863 by purchasing, among other items, 89 bunks, 100 mattresses and pillows, and 200 pillow cases. The structure seemed to be plagued by fire. In May 1862, before the CSN occupied the Gibbons House, an adjacent building containing part of the city gas works caught fire and caused an unreported amount of damage to the hotel. In November 1863, fire damaged a floor of the Gibbons House but evidently caused little or no harm to CSN patients or property. In mid–February 1864, fire destroyed much of the building, but CSN furniture, bedding, and medicines were largely saved, and patients were moved to the Confederate army's General Hospital No. 1 in Savannah. It appears that this fire marked the end of the CSN's use of the Gibbons House. The capacity of the Gibbons House hospital is difficult to determine, but it had 37 patients on October 1, 1863.[28]

The CSN then rented a house to serve as a hospital from about March through August 1864 at the corner of West Broad and Zubly Streets, only a block or so from the Gibbons House, at $180 a month. It appears that use of the building lasted for several months and overlapped with a return to the City Hospital, because starting no later than May 1864, the CSN began to rent the latter at $200 per month and to pay for gas provided to the building.[29]

Among patients evidently treated at the City Hospital, this time by CSN personnel, were USN crewmen injured during the capture of USS *Water Witch* in June 1864. Acting Assistant Surgeon W.H. Pierson, USN, described the facility as "devoid of some of the luxuries which may be found in Northern Hospitals" but "airy and comfortable." Patients there, said Pierson, "received every care and comfort which the somewhat limited resources of the country well admitted." The hospital was under the charge of Surgeon Richard W. Jeffery, CSN, who with his assistant surgeons, treated Pierson with "gentlemanly consideration." (The CSN medical personnel serving at the hospital at about the same time were Assistant Surgeons William S. Stoakley and John B. Rutherford.) Another Union prisoner, Paymaster Luther Guiteau Billings, described the hospital as "a most commodious dwelling which faced one of the numerous squares in that beautiful old city." Billings was probably referring to the South Commons; the former hospitals on Broad Street did not face a square.[30]

The Savannah Naval Hospital—which probably dated from about July 1863, when the Gibbons House was rented for that purpose—admitted 128 patients during the first three quarters of 1863, discharged 81, had four die, and had 37 remaining on October 1 (the remaining six deserted). During the year ending October 1, 1864, the hospital admitted 394 patients, discharged 270, and had 15 die. During the first quarter of 1864, the hospital employed six civilians: one ward matron, one nurse, and four part-time laundresses. One patient during that quarter was Surgeon Henry W.M. Washington, CSN. During the third quarter of 1864, civilian employees included one steward, one matron, one nurse, one part-time cook, and six part-time laundresses. It has not been determined whether any of the CSN hospitals in Savannah used an ambulance. At times, civilians were paid to transport patients or their baggage to the hospital.[31]

The structure then called the City Hospital served after the war as the site of Candler Hospital and the now-defunct Savannah Law School. It is now Ruskin Hall of the Savannah School of Art and Design. The bad luck afflicting the Gibbons House culminated in late January 1865, the month after Union troops occupied Savannah. A building near West Broad and Zubly Streets caught fire and ignited munitions stored nearby. Several lives were lost, and a large swath of structures in the area—including the Gibbons House and presumably the building at West Broad and Zubly also used as a CSN hospital—was totally destroyed.[32]

Wilmington and Smithville, North Carolina

The two naval hospitals on North Carolina's Cape Fear River appear to have been established during the first half of 1864 and were evidently managed by the same medical officers. Wilmington, about 30 miles from the mouth of the river, had suffered an epidemic of yellow fever during the summer of 1862, during which one of the CSN medical officers stationed there, Surgeon James W.B. Greenhow, "although not required to stay, did so as a volunteer, and never once slackened his exertions" in treating patients. Wilmington had

10. Hospitals

yards where naval vessels were built, and it became the South's major blockade-running port during the second half of the war. As late as December 1863, a private physician, William H. Hill, was paid to visit and treat patients at the Wilmington Navy Yard. The town's naval hospital was situated on Chestnut Street, between Water and Front Streets, and was directed in December 1864 by Passed Assistant Surgeon John W. Sandford, Jr., who was assisted by Assistant Surgeon Robert C. Kuykendall. Little is known about the facility, other than the fact that it admitted 135 patients and discharged 90 during the second and third quarters of 1864.[33]

Located near the mouth of the river, Smithville (now called Southport) was the site of Confederate Fort Pender—originally Fort Johnston—which helped guard the approach to Wilmington. The ironclad *North Carolina* and other vessels were sent to the Smithville area to assist in that task. There was also thought to be a naval depot in the area. Starting no later than January 1864, the CSN rented a house, at $100 per month, in Smithville from Mrs. A.C. Everitt for use as a hospital. Most of the vouchers for rent or supplies for the hospital were signed by Passed Assistant Surgeon Sandford, although at least two were signed by Surgeon Greenhow as fleet surgeon of the North Carolina Squadron. In April 1864, OMS chief Spotswood mentioned the upcoming need for the Smithville hospital to have a medical officer with the grade of surgeon, but it is unclear whether such an officer was ever assigned. Details about the hospital's capacity or operations have not been found.[34]

Others Hospitals

Confederate records mention a naval hospital on Roanoke Island, North Carolina, in 1861, and in Charlotte—associated with the Naval Works there and manned by Surgeon Charles H. Williamson—in 1863. The fortifications at Drewry's Bluff, Virginia, whose personnel included Confederate marines and men from the CSN, including medical officers, were reported to have "several subterranean hospitals for the reception of the wounded." Hospitals served by naval medical officers also existed at Fort Fisher and Post of Arkansas, but whether those facilities were managed by the CSN is unknown. Little or no additional information about these facilities has been found. Medical officers served and received medical supplies at various naval stations not mentioned above, but whether naval hospitals were ever established at those locales has not been determined.[35]

In June 1862, Spotswood dispatched Surgeon Richard W. Jeffery to Greensboro, North Carolina, to determine the cost of establishing a naval hospital there. Neither the results of Jeffery's mission nor information about the proposed facility have been found.[36]

Hospital Ships

The CSN employed a small number of vessels as floating hospitals or transports for the sick and wounded. One that might qualify as such was "a long flat-boat" attached to the floating battery that participated in the bombardment of Fort Sumter in April 1861. The battery, which had to be towed into position, was designed and commanded by Lieutenant John R. Hamilton, CSN, but the hospital section was directed by civilian physician (and later army surgeon) Columbus Davega, with assistance by a Dr. Doucing, who has not been further identified.[37]

The most is known about CSS *St. Philip*, formerly *Star of the West*, under which name it made an unsuccessful attempt to carry Federal reinforcements and supplies from New York to Fort Sumter in January 1861. The vessel was later captured by Confederate forces and used as a naval recruiting, receiving, and hospital ship at New Orleans. One observer described the vessel as "large, airy, and furnishing comfortable sleeping quarters at night for at least 1000 men." The vessel was removed before the loss of New Orleans and eventually sunk as a river obstruction. Surgeon Lewis W. Minor, as surgeon of the New Orleans Station, and Surgeon Daniel B. Conrad appear to have shared responsibility for the hospital functions of CSS *St. Philip*; a register of patients shows 130 admissions between September 1861 and April 1862. Some CSN patients from vessels stationed at New Orleans were sent to

10. Hospitals

Charity Hospital in the city. By April 24, 1862, Minor's responsibilities for *St. Philip* appear to have ended, since Captain William C. Whittle, commanding the New Orleans Station, told Minor that there was "no duty that I am aware of for you to perform here now" and that Minor should avoid being captured by the oncoming enemy.[38]

The steamers *Samuel Orr* and *Patton* were reportedly used as Confederate hospitals on the Tennessee River when Fort Henry was surrendered to Union forces in February 1862, but it is unclear whether they were considered CSN vessels. *Patton* had 16 men aboard when surrendered, but how many were patients was not reported. The steamer *Kanawha Valley* was a Confederate watch or hospital boat that was wrecked in a storm near Island No. 10 in the Mississippi River on April 1 and 2, 1862; its association with the CSN is also unknown. The CSN had a hospital ship (name unknown) near Savannah in October 1861, but nothing else is known about the vessel.[39]

In May 1864, CSN officials planned to convert CSS *Patrick Henry* into a hospital ship for the James River Squadron. The vessel was serving as home to the Confederate States Naval Academy, but a Federal advance under Major General Benjamin F. Butler that month prompted the assignment of the academy's midshipmen to various defensive positions. In September 1864, classes on *Patrick Henry* resumed. Whether the vessel had actually ever served as a hospital ship has not been determined.[40]

* * *

Unless abandoned USN hospitals were available, as was the case at Pensacola and Norfolk, the CSN used civilian hospitals and, in several instances, established its own in preexisting structures. Hospitals attended by naval surgeons tended to be associated with squadrons—as was the case in Richmond, Mobile, Charleston, Savannah, and Wilmington—and employed local civilians as attendants. Hospitals might also exist at naval batteries and fortifications, such as those at Drewry's Bluff, Fort Fisher, and Post of Arkansas. The CSN's medical corps devoted considerable resources to its hospitals, a circumstance driven by high rates of illness rather than by battle or other injuries.

– 11 –

Treating the Sick

Naval surgeons were called upon to treat many different illnesses and injuries. Data concerning the frequency of various diagnoses throughout the CSN were undoubtedly collected by the OMS but most did not survive the war. Because complete summary statistics are not available, it is not possible to know exactly how prevalent specific aliments were among Confederate naval or marine corps personnel or whether certain subsets of sailors or marines might have been disproportionately affected by specific disorders. Hospital records provide some information about patients—including their self-reported age and country of origin—common medical conditions, and treatments. Data are particularly sparse on ailments that were not serious enough to necessitate hospitalization.

Consolidated data for January through September 1863 show 6,122 admissions to hospitals (including sickbays), plus 135 patients remaining hospitalized from the previous quarter. If it is assumed that there were about 6,000 officers and men in the navy and marine corps, there was slightly more than one admission, on average, per member of the navy and marine corps during those nine months. Such a rate could be fairly benign if sickness were evenly distributed in place and time, but it might also compromise the navy's fighting efficiency if illness were localized among specific squadrons or stations or occurred at about the same time, especially with long hospitalizations. Among those admissions, there were 5,766 hospital discharges, 59 deaths (about 1.0 percent mortality), and 28 desertions; the remaining patients were still hospitalized when the data were reported. For the year starting October 1863, admissions dropped to 1,995, with 1,410 discharges and 69 deaths (3.5 percent mortality). Thus, although the death rate

11. Treating the Sick

increased—for reasons that are unclear—the rate of admission dropped markedly.[1]

The changes occurred after OMS chief Spotswood recommended relocating the Mobile Squadron to a spot where he thought malaria would be less troublesome. In fact, if the same nine months (January through September) are compared for 1863 and 1864, admissions at the Mobile Station plummeted from 2,219 to 274, while deaths dropped from 13 to eight. Although Spotswood reported that illness in the James River Squadron was more problematic in the summer and fall of 1864 compared with 1863, the number of admissions for the Richmond Station, which comprised more than just the James River Squadron, actually dropped from 1,123 for January through September 1863 to 768 for the same months in 1864.[2]

Partial records for CSN hospitalizations are available for the hospital ship *St. Philip* stationed at New Orleans (records for December 1861–April 1862) and that city's Charity Hospital (records for November 1861), both of which admitted patients from the Mississippi River Squadron; CSS *General Polk* of the Mississippi River Squadron (records for November 1861–May 1862); CSS *Atlanta*, operating out of Savannah (records for December 1862–June 1863); and CSS *Gaines* of the Mobile Squadron (records for May 1862–August 1863). The pooled data account for about 370 patients. The youngest were 13 years old and rated as boys; a few others in their teens were midshipmen. Most patients were in their 20s and 30s, and the oldest were 60 years of age. Almost all hospitalized commissioned or warrant officers had been born in one of the seceding or border states. In contrast, 41 percent of *Gaines*'s hospitalized seamen had been born in Ireland, 17 percent in continental Europe, 14 percent in a seceding state, 9 percent in England, 8 percent in a state remaining in the Union, and 5 percent in Scotland. On *Gaines*, 11 of the 177 hospitalized seamen for whom a birthplace was reported were said to be from Manila, in the Philippine Islands.[3]

From the medicines allowed officially by the OMS, it appears that treatment was based on allopathic principles rather than on one or more of the sectarian doctrines of the time. The OMS evidently did not require particular diagnoses to be handled in a standard fashion, so medical officers could prescribe as they saw fit, within the confines—which could be significant—of the available medicines and instruments. A USN surgeon described a medical officer's situation, which surely applied to the CSN as well: "The life of every physician in practice is subject to vexations from the nature of his profession. On ship-board, and particularly when he is at sea, he is still more liable to annoyance from the inconvenience he must of necessity suffer from his constrained position, his not having at command the space required to practice successfully, or such remedies and appliances as can be had on land."[4]

Malaria

Malaria was the malady that caused the most difficulty in the CSN. The disease, caused by a unicellular parasite, was not then known to be transmitted by mosquitoes. Instead, practitioners noted that the illness was associated with marshes, decomposing vegetable matter, and warm weather and postulated that such conditions generated noxious emanations (miasmas) that caused disease. In fact, physicians of the time used the term *malaria* (bad air) to describe the miasmas rather than the associated illness, which was often called intermittent or periodic fever—or in the official CSN nomenclature of disease, *febris intermittens*.[5]

In November 1863, OMS chief Spotswood reported that officers and men at Mobile "suffered exceedingly from exposure to the malarial causes that exist there during the summer and fall months." He recommended moving the Mobile Squadron's anchorage away from the marshes by the city to the opposite side of Mobile Bay, where the conditions were much healthier. Assistant Surgeon Osborn S. Iglehart of CSS *Gaines*, part of the Mobile Squadron, documented the seasonal variation in malaria cases. Although no month was free of malaria, the number of sickbay admissions for malaria increased from 11 in June 1862 to 29 the following month. August and September 1862 saw 49 and 33 admissions for malaria, with the crest occurring in October, with 55 of 73 admissions being attributed

11. Treating the Sick

to malaria. The next most common admission diagnosis in October 1862 was rheumatism, with four admissions. Malaria admissions for *Gaines* dropped to 10 in November 1862. Iglehart's known records for *Gaines* do not extend beyond August 1863, but in that month, there were 112 admissions for malaria among 80 different patients. Thus, about 62 percent of the vessel's complement of 130 officers and men were ill enough with the disease during the month to be admitted to sickbay, and with an average stay of about five days, malaria had a substantial effect on manpower.[6]

In November 1864, Spotswood reported malaria as a particular problem, especially at Savannah and Charleston. At Savannah, said Spotswood, "the fevers have been marked with unusual severity on board of vessels that, from the nature of the duty, had their crews necessarily exposed to the action of the malaria of the freshwater rivers and swamps bordering the rice fields." According to Spotswood, changing the location of the vessels reduced the problem. Records of CSS *Atlanta*, based at Savannah, show 75 admissions for malaria among 40 patients during a span of about seven months. *Atlanta* had a complement of about 145, and one of its crew was admitted nine times to sickbay during that time with a diagnosis of malaria.[7]

The James River Squadron suffered from malaria in summer and fall 1864 because of a prolonged dry spell, "causing the river to fall lower than ever, and thus generating a greater amount of malaria" because of greater expanses of stagnant water. The reaction of the squadron's flag officer, John K. Mitchell, was to move the vessels' anchorage away from Boulware's Landing, which he described as "particularly unhealthy, owing to an extensive marsh on the south side of the river." Spotswood and a group of surgeons investigating the squadron's health problems recommended measures that would serve to "fortify" crews against malarial attacks, such as providing ventilation and shade on the ironclads, allowing exercise on shore, obtaining fresh fruits and vegetables, and issuing the whiskey ration with hot coffee in the morning.[8]

Malaria was also problematic at New Orleans. Among eight CSN patients treated at Charity Hospital in New Orleans in November

The Confederate Navy Medical Corps

1861, five had malaria, two had syphilis, and one had asthma. Among 130 admissions to hospital ship *St. Philip* at New Orleans in 1861 and 1862, 48 were for malaria.⁹

Quinine (as quinine sulfate) was generally considered to be the treatment of choice for malaria, but it was relatively expensive even before the war because its manufacture required relatively complex laboratory procedures. Quinine could also cause troublesome adverse effects and did not always work. Furthermore, there was doubt about whether it could prevent malaria, not just lessen or eradicate its symptoms. Quinine dosages could vary widely and were often adjusted according to a patient's response and the timing of his or her chills and fevers. A typical quinine regimen for treating malaria might consist of 15–20 grains (about 975–1,300 milligrams) during a day, in divided doses.¹⁰

Assistant Surgeon Iglehart of the Mobile Squadron prescribed quinine regularly to treat the symptoms of malaria. On August 4, 1863, he recorded, "By order of Admiral [Franklin] Buchanan [commander of the Mobile Squadron and Station], under my direction,

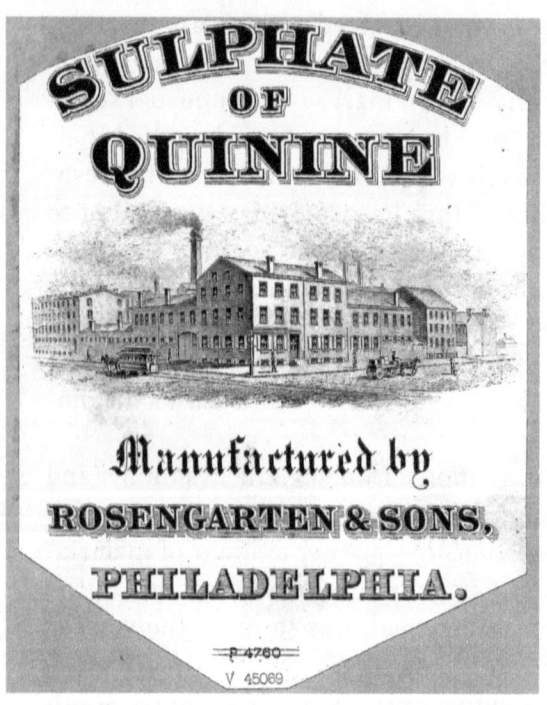

Label design, probably from the late 1800s, for quinine made by Rosengarten and Sons. The company was one of only two American firms, both based in Philadelphia, that manufactured quinine during the Civil War. The Confederacy obtained the drug, which was also made in Europe, through smuggling, capture, and blockade-running. Quinine's price, especially in the South, increased substantially during the war (author's collection).

11. Treating the Sick

whiskey is administered to certain of the crew each morning, mixed with quinine." Iglehart's recipe called for three avoirdupois ounces of quinine in ten gallons of whiskey, with a dose (one fluid ounce) of the mixture containing about 66 milligrams (just over a grain) of quinine. (Mixing quinine with whiskey tended to mask the drug's extreme bitterness and encourage sailors to accept the medication.) Iglehart was apparently trying to prevent malaria, as suggested by the large amount of whiskey (enough for about 1,300 doses) and the size of the quinine dose, which was much smaller than that used to treat the active disease. Iglehart's action was probably the basis of one report that quinine was given with the spirit ration in the Mobile Squadron during summer 1863 in an unsuccessful—and ultimately abandoned—attempt to prevent malaria. Iglehart's own reporting of the results of his trial has not been found, but because the quinine dosage that he used was only a quarter to a half of what other physicians were prescribing for the same purpose, failure would not have been surprising.[11]

Because of quinine's limitations, prewar practitioners tried malaria treatments that might prove helpful while being cheaper and safer. That quest was continued during the war by the Confederate army medical department, whose chief, Surgeon General Samuel Preston Moore, encouraged surgeons to investigate and use remedies derived from indigenous plants. Although there is no good indication that OMS chief Spotswood aggressively adopted the same course, his medical purveying department did have to deal with quinine's scarcity and price.[12]

One option was to use cinchona bark—the raw material from which quinine was made—rather than quinine itself. OMS apothecary Robert Lecky purchased Calisaya bark, a variety of cinchona, and used a relatively simple process to make compound tincture of Peruvian bark for distribution to ships and hospitals. The bark had some of the medicinal qualities of quinine and was less expensive, but it was inferior to quinine for the treatment of malaria. (Blockade-runners probably did not bring much cinchona bark to the South because it was much bulkier than quinine and unlikely to produce similar profits.) Lecky also purchased boneset and issued it as an extract. The boneset or thoroughwort plant grew in the South and was thought by some practitioners to be useful in malaria, but a standard drug textbook cautioned that "the general experience, however, is not in its favor in that complaint." Boneset was among the many indigenous plants used by the Confederate army, but the extent to which it was used in the CSN is unknown.[13]

A medication perhaps intended as a quinine substitute was extract of hemp. That formulation, made from the plant *Cannabis indica*—considered to be a variety of *C. sativa* (hemp or marijuana)—was not on the army's or navy's standard supply table. Nevertheless, it was purchased for use on CSS *Patrick Henry* in November 1861 from the Richmond drug wholesaler Purcell, Ladd and Company. Known for its sedative and other properties, *C. indica* was commonly called Indian hemp, but that moniker also applied to *Apocynum cannabinum*, a plant native to North American that had been reported in 1859 to be an effective remedy for malaria by Peterfield Trent, a Richmond physician and wartime surgeon with the Second Regiment of Virginia State Reserves. Medicinal preparations of *C. indica* and *A. cannabinum* were rarely if ever prescribed by Confederate surgeons, but the known tendency for the two species to be confused with each other raises the possibility that the *C. indica* extract was thought to be made from *A. cannabinum* when purchased by the CSN and meant for trial as an antimalarial treatment.[14]

One treatment in popular favor was a solution of potassium arsenite, known formally as liquor potassae arsenitis and popularly as Fowler's solution. One professor of medicine believed that arsenic—one medicinal form of which was Fowler's solution—was "adequate to the cure of intermittent fever in a very great majority of cases, and, indeed, that few will resist it if judiciously employed." Assistant Surgeon Robert R. Gibbes, while serving on CSS *Fingal* in mid–1862, reported that "most cases responded well to a good diet and administration of quinine and Fowler's 'solution.'" Fowler's solution was included among medicines allowed on CSN vessels and in CSN hospitals.[15]

In July 1861, Southern newspapers published a malaria remedy advocated by Surgeon Dinwiddie B. Phillips, CSN. When Phillips had been in the USN, he had occasion to administer "a negro remedy," raw corn meal (from *Zea mays*, or Indian corn), for malaria and reported that "in the hot stages of intermittent fever, it may be given in ice water, and will be found to relieve thirst, and cool the skin sooner and better than any remedy I know." Phillips's reports had been published in a medical journal in 1857 and 1858, but the 1861 newspaper account added new remarks that Phillips probably provided himself: the remedy could also take the form of a "tea made of fodder" and could also be used "in all stages of the disease without the slightest evil effects." Both corn meal and fodder tea—the latter made from the blades of *Zea mays*—had been recommended in 1852 by at least one other author. A trial of fodder tea was conducted by a Confederate army surgeon at Howard's Grove Hospital in Richmond, but whether Phillips or any other CSN surgeon prescribed corn meal or fodder tea for malaria has not been determined.[16]

Diarrhea and Dysentery

Diarrhea was a fairly common ailment among sailors and generally thought, at the time, to result from bowel inflammation. Diarrhea, accompanied by blood and mucus in the stool and pain when defecating, might be diagnosed as dysentery. Food that was difficult to digest, spoiled, or poorly prepared could cause diarrhea, as could any number of infectious agents.

When Assistant Surgeon Iglehart treated a sailor suffering from diarrhea on May 26, 1862, he prescribed lead acetate, probably as an astringent, which would constrict tissues and reduce bowel secretions, and opium to reduce the frequency of watery stools. However, noted Igelhart, "The difficulty in treating these cases is owing to the want of proper medicines." On January 2, 1863, when treating a patient with dysentery, Iglehart again administered lead acetate and opium but complained, "Medicine has but little beneficial effect, without change of diet, at this stage of the disease. Requires a change of diet, which I am unable to give him." Iglehart did not indicate which drugs he was lacking or the type of diet he would have ordered.[17]

Patients with diarrhea or dysentery on CSS *General Polk* and CSS *Atlanta* were often treated with tannic acid, probably as an astringent, and opium, by itself or as a component of Dover's powder, which also contained powder of ipecacuanha and potassium sulfate. Sometimes the initial treatment for diarrhea was a laxative, in the form of castor oil or mercury pills, to clear the bowel of noxious material thought to be causing inflammation, followed by opium.[18]

Rheumatism

The term *rheumatism*, as used by naval surgeons, was nonspecific and seemed a catch-all for various pains around the joints. A popular medical dictionary of the era defined rheumatism as "a kind of shifting phlegmasia [inflammation] or neuralgia [pain along the course of nerves], sometimes seated in the muscles, sometimes in the parts surrounding the joints; and at others, within them." Although practitioners could describe rheumatism as being muscular, articular, or synovial—and further as acute or chronic—standard naval nomenclature did not allow such specificity. According to that nomenclature, rheumatism was among diseases of the fibrous (connective-tissue), muscular, and osseous (skeletal) systems. If the disorder could not be determined as being centered in either the bones or joints, then the naval surgeon had to call the ailment either rheumatism or podagra (pain in the foot or gout). Ailments called rheumatism were among the more common complaints treated by CSN surgeons. Many cases of Civil War rheumatism were probably acute rheumatic fever, known today to be caused by a streptococcal infection. In other instances, rheumatism may have been a reactive arthritis following venereal infections or dysentery.[19]

In managing rheumatism, potassium iodide, a popular treatment of the day, was routinely prescribed by Assistant Surgeon Iglehart of CSS *Gaines* and on occasions by the medical officers of CSS *Atlanta*. On the latter vessel and on CSS *General Polk*, the most common treatment was an alcoholic preparation of colchicum seed, often used at the time for gout. (Colchicine, which is derived from colchicum, has been used for the same indication in more modern times.) Colchicum was likely to cause gastrointestinal upset, so on *Atlanta*, it was sometimes given in combination with calcined magnesia. Naval surgeons also prescribed opium pills, Dover's powder, or a liniment to manage the pain of rheumatism.[20]

Catarrh

Men were commonly diagnosed with catarrh, a nonspecific term that indicated an increased discharge of mucus from the air passages; such patients were frequently described by medical officers having as a chest cold or head cold. Treatment often included Dover's powder, which had expectorant (secretion-loosening) and cough-suppressant properties. The same effects were likely produced by mixtures used by Assistant Surgeon Iglehart of CSS *Gaines* (syrup of squill and camphorated tincture of opium [paregoric]) and Assistant Surgeon Robert R. Gibbes of CSS *Atlanta* (syrup of seneka, antimonial wine, gum arabic, and tincture of opium). Catarrh may occasionally have been treated with tincture of lobelia, made from a plant indigenous to North America. Tincture of lobelia did not appear in the CSN standard supply table but was mentioned by the Confederate army as useful for its expectorant properties and was purchased by the OMS from Purcell, Ladd and Company. Some physicians used it in asthma, catarrh, "and other laryngeal and pectoral affections."[21]

Yellow Fever

Yellow fever—known now to be caused by a virus and transmitted by virus-carrying mosquitoes—was probably more feared than malaria because of its deadliness and the intense suffering it caused. The disease was associated with the same sorts of conditions thought to engender malaria, especially in the presence of poor sanitation. Quarantines were usually imposed, but there was no general agreement on how the disease should be treated. Surgeon James W.B.

Greenhow cared for patients during the 1862 yellow fever epidemic in Wilmington, and the disease ravaged the small crew of CSS *Florida* in August 1862, which at the time had no surgeons. *Florida*'s commander, Lieutenant John N. Maffitt, administered to the sick until he too was stricken, and local medical assistance was provided while the vessel was anchored off of Cuba. Yellow fever probably contributed to suffering even in men never infected with the illness, because quarantines and fear of docking at afflicted ports disrupted the flow of medical and other supplies delivered by blockade-runners.[22]

Passed Assistant Surgeon Robert R. Gibbes noted sporadic cases of yellow fever in Charleston starting around August 8, 1864, but cases became "fearfully fatal and epidemic" in mid–September. Between October 11 and 26, 19 men died at the Charleston Naval Hospital of the disease, including Assistant Surgeon David E. Ewart. On October 26, Gibbes developed chills, nausea and vomiting, headache, extreme pain in the lumbar region, and intense fever—all of which convinced him that he too had contracted the disease. By November 5, Gibbes had recovered sufficiently to care for himself.[23]

Smallpox

Smallpox was feared because of its severity and communicability, a fact well illustrated by an anecdote recorded by Assistant Surgeon Gibbes. A fellow medical officer, who had never seen the disease, suspected a case of smallpox on CSS *Savannah* (then stationed at Savannah) and informed the squadron and station commander, Captain Josiah Tatnall, who informed the city's health officer. That official, who himself had never seen a case, declared that smallpox was indeed the culprit, and the patient was quickly placed in a tent, along with an attendant, on a flatboat away from CSS *Savannah*. Gibbes, who had attended many cases of smallpox, visited the patient and quickly surmised that he was suffering from psoriasis rather than smallpox. The patient himself had contracted smallpox as a youth and knew his current affliction was not that disease.

11. Treating the Sick

Nevertheless, said Gibbes, the local populace looked at crewmembers as if they were infected with the plague, and CSS *Savannah* was placed under quarantine, with the patient sent to a pest house ashore. The patient was well when next visited by Gibbes, who convinced the health officer that smallpox was not present, and the vessel's quarantine was lifted.[24]

Smallpox appears only rarely in CSN records, possibly because naval surgeons were largely successful in seeing that all recruits were vaccinated. Sailors with known or suspected smallpox were sometimes cared for in army hospitals that could properly isolate the patients and offer treatment. Such patients from the Richmond Naval Hospital and nearby Drewry's Bluff were sent to a Richmond army hospital during December 1862, during a smallpox outbreak in the city. For the period of October 1862 to mid–January 1863, Surgeon William A. Carrington, Inspector of Hospitals and Acting Medical Director in Richmond, reported that 774 patients had been admitted to the city's army hospitals with smallpox and that 284 had died. Carrington considered the mortality rate (almost 37 percent) from the "obnoxious and loathsome disease" to be "very great." The dread of smallpox, it seems, was well-founded.[25]

Vaccination necessitated the collection of fluid ("lymph") or scabs from the lesions of people or cows with cowpox or from people with smallpox. After some manipulation, that material, called vaccine matter, was then introduced into small openings made in the skin of the person being vaccinated. USN surgeons could requisition vaccine matter from the Brooklyn naval laboratory, but exactly how CNS surgeons obtained it is unclear. They may have purchased it from blockade-runners or from firms selling medical supplies. Local practitioners or medical officers themselves may also have collected and prepared vaccine matter.[26]

Vaccination was not always effective in preventing smallpox, and it could produce unexpected illness or unusual lesions at or beyond the vaccination site. That phenomenon, called spurious vaccination, was usually attributed to impure or tainted vaccine matter. Nevertheless, it is likely that the overall effect of vaccination on the health of CSN personnel was positive.[27]

Sexually Transmitted Diseases

Naval surgeons treated sexually transmitted diseases, with syphilis being much more commonly diagnosed than gonorrhea. Syphilitic penile chancres were routinely treated with topical applications of silver nitrate, which were intended to cauterize the lesions and promote healing. Lesions were sometimes painted with "black wash," which was made by mixing mild chloride of mercury (calomel) with a solution of calcium hydroxide in water (lime water). Passed Assistant Surgeon Charles E. Lining of CSS *Shenandoah* reported that the first crewmember to die during a long cruise succumbed to a presumed case of constitutional syphilis.[28]

Assistant Surgeon Iglehart diagnosed acute syphilis in a patient with an ulcerating penile chancre. He cauterized the sore (possibly with silver nitrate or zinc chloride) but noted, "Should be touched with nitric acid, but there is none in the ship" and, a week later, "Shall apply nitric acid as soon as can obtain it." Iglehart did not describe treating the patient with nitric acid until 10 days after he initially mentioned lacking it and five days after he transferred a patient to the Mobile Naval Hospital. His not having nitric acid on hand in CSS *Gaines*—vessels with a full supply of allowable medical supplies would have some—and not acquiring any from the hospital during the transfer suggest that the OMS had difficulty purchasing or transporting it. Nitric acid, in fact, was in short supply in the Confederacy. Not only did it have medicinal uses, but the War Department's Ordnance Bureau also needed it to manufacture fulminate of mercury, the explosive in percussion caps, and the Confederacy's Military Telegraph Office needed it for its wet-cell batteries. The army's Columbia, South Carolina, medical laboratory started manufacturing nitric acid the year after Iglehart complained about its unavailability.[29]

The one patient diagnosed with gonorrhea in Assistant Surgeon Iglehart's journal received urethral injections of a mixture of zinc sulfate and tincture of opium. Assistant Surgeon Robert J. Freeman on CSS *General Polk* treated a crewmember who had a urethral

11. Treating the Sick

stricture and painful urinary retention, possibly due to a gonorrheal infection. Freeman had no instrument small enough to pass the obstruction, but he enabled the patient to urinate after introducing and withdrawing the stylet (a thin metal stiffener) ordinarily used with a gum-rubber catheter. Freeman was supposed to have an assortment of metallic bougies, small-caliber curved rods to dilate the urethra, but had to borrow some from one of the squadron's gunboats. After successfully passing the smallest one past the stricture, Freeman gradually increased the bougie size and was able to discharge the patient from sickbay after about a two-week stay; use of the bougies, however, continued after that.[30]

Scurvy

Physicians of the Civil War era knew that scurvy, known now to result from vitamin C deficiency, could be prevented by a diet containing sufficient amounts of fruits and vegetables, particularly if fresh. The weekly standard ration of the CSN included components that, in the right proportions, might help prevent scurvy—a half-pound of raisins or dried fruit and a half-pound of pickles or cranberries—but the extent to which actual diets contained those items is unknown. With the exception of commerce raiders and blockade-runners, most CSN vessels did not go on extended cruises and thus had relatively frequent opportunities to dock at ports where such foodstuffs, if available, could be obtained. Raphael Semmes, captain of the cruiser *Sumter*, described scurvy on his vessel and the efforts to control it with fresh provisions, and Passed Assistant Surgeon Charles E. Lining of the commerce raider *Shenandoah* feared scurvy during a prolonged cruise. Although Assistant Surgeon Iglehart noted symptoms of scurvy in a CSS *Gaines* patient with fever, scurvy generally did not seem problematic in that vessel, at least among men admitted to sickbay. Modern research revealed signs suggestive of scurvy in skeletal remains of Confederate sailors and marines at a Charleston cemetery, but the investigators were unable to make a definite diagnosis.[31]

Seasickness

Seasickness was not among the maladies reported by crewmembers admitted to the sickbay of CSS *General Polk*, *Atlanta*, or *Gaines*. Those vessels were stationed on the Mississippi River, the area around Savannah, and Mobile Bay, respectively, so perhaps waters were not turbulent enough to cause seasickness or sailors did not get ill enough to be mentioned in surgeons' journals. On the other hand, Robert R. Gibbes, during his brief service with the South Carolina navy, was present on a cruise of the guard boat *Gordon* as that vessel ventured about 30 miles outside of Charleston on a rough sea. He was called on to attend multiple ailing volunteers, who were evidently unaccustomed to life on the sea and said they would certainly die from seasickness unless he could help them.[32]

Gibbes's general advice for seasickness echoed that of other naval surgeons. In particular, afflicted persons should not dwell on their misery but go about their business. They should go on deck, get plenty of fresh air; look at the sky or horizon (rather than at the ship's rigging), and not avoid food. In fact, said one surgeon, highly flavored food—for example, salt fish, boiled ham, ginger cakes, or preserved ginger—could be helpful, as could aromatic drinks, such as tea, coffee, wine, rum, or brandy. "Gibbes recommended that a meal should be preceded by ingesting a glass of strong vinegar and some biscuit or bread."[33]

There were no tried-and-true remedies for seasickness. Treatments considered useful included ingesting ice water or "acidulated drinks"—perhaps made my adding lemon juice or vinegar to water—and opiates. Small doses of creosote might also be used.[34]

Other Ailments

Tooth decay was extremely common—skeletal remains of Confederate sailors and marines revealed an average of almost seven cavities per mouth—so naval surgeons undoubtedly spent time using the tooth-extracting instruments issued to them. Passed Assistant

11. Treating the Sick

Surgeon Lining recorded "efforts to pull the mate's tooth" in his CSS *Shenandoah* journal.[35]

Perhaps less expected on *Shenandoah* was the discovery of bedbugs, against which "war" was declared. Bedbugs, and the bites they inflicted, were supposedly common on old ships, but mentions of them on Civil War vessels are rare.[36]

The Spirit Ration

Although the spirit ration was suspended in November 1863 because whiskey was too difficult to procure, senior CSN surgeons were convinced that the ration—which was considered separately from medicinal alcohol—had value. When asked in August 1864 to recommend measures to reduce malarial illness in the James River Squadron, Surgeons William B. Sinclair, James F. Harrison, and William F. Carrington were "decidedly of the opinion that the whiskey ration be issued to the men with hot coffee given every morning at an early hour." OMS chief Spotswood expanded on the recommendation by explaining that the coffee and whiskey would help to counteract "the effects of the damp and chilling drafts so prevalent on all fresh-water courses and malarial regions at the dawn of day." All four officers had served in the USN, where the spirit ration was a long-standing tradition inherited from the British navy. Whiskey was believed by some to help fortify men exposed to hard work or harsh weather. Thus, when the spirit ration was abolished in 1862 in the Federal navy—in part because it supposedly contributed to drunkenness—USN commander Charles Wilkes argued for its usefulness, especially for crews exposed to "fatiguing and exposed service." Highly respected army officers of the Civil War also believed in the fortifying properties of whiskey. Surgeon Jonathan Letterman of the U.S. Army, recommended that troops arriving in camp after a march be given a gill of whiskey in a canteen three-fourths filled with water, and Confederate army surgeon J. J Chisolm said that a dram of whiskey—a gill was probably meant, since a dram was less than a teaspoonful—helped to sustain health in soldiers without tents and exposed to "the drenching rains or the heavy nightly dews."[37]

The Confederate Navy Medical Corps

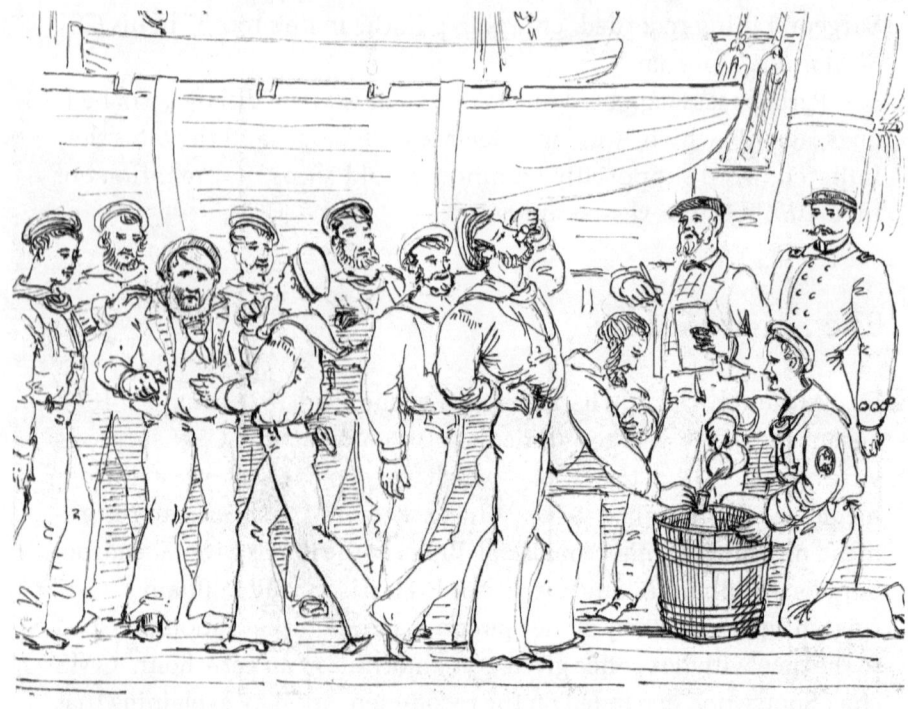

Sketch by Charles Ellery Stedman of Union sailors receiving their spirit ration. The ration was discontinued by the USN in 1862 and by the CSN in 1863, yet many CSN surgeons believed that it was medically beneficial (Civil War Photograph Collection, vol. 14, MOLLUS-MASS, USAHEC).

Issuing whiskey to sailors was also rationalized on the grounds that it encouraged recruitment and that the threat of withholding it helped to maintain discipline. Nevertheless, having liquor aboard and not under a surgeon's immediate control—as stores of medical alcohol were—could be problematic. Much drunkenness ensued when crewmembers of CSS *Shenandoah* surreptitiously removed more than 50 gallons of rum from a barrel and when liquor was brought aboard against orders. On another occasion, wine on that vessel was stolen from the dispensary. After *Shenandoah*'s officers and men learned in August 1865 of the collapse of the Confederate States—the vessel was in the Pacific Ocean at the time—the captain asked Passed Assistant Surgeon Lining whether the services of contract surgeon Frederick J. McNulty could be dispensed with.

11. Treating the Sick

McNulty, said Lining, was "drunk on every occasion," got into quarrels, and challenged a lieutenant to a duel.[38]

* * *

Medical officers devoted considerable effort to treating sickness. Malaria was, by far, the most troublesome illness and accounted for surgeons spending much of their time caring for stricken patients and suggesting ways of preventing the disease. Efforts to provide optimal care were sometimes hampered—especially on vessels, on which resources were necessarily limited in range and quantity—by inadequate supplies of medicines or instruments.

– 12 –

Rendering Judgments

Surgeons in the CSN spent some portion of their time examining men and supplies and being scrutinized themselves. In some cases, their opinion was sought not because of their medical aptitude but because of their standing as naval officers.

Examination of Recruits

Naval medical officers were assigned to recruiting stations called naval rendezvous, where they examined men applying for enlisted positions in the navy. The USN guidance for such officers stated:

> They will cause each recruit to be stripped of all his clothes, to move about, exercise his limbs in their presence, in order to ascertain whether he has free use of them; that his chest is ample, that his hearing, vision and speech are good, that he has no tumors, ulcerated or extensively cicatrized legs, rupture, chronic cutaneous affection, or other disorder or infirmity, mental or physical, which may render him unfit for the active duties of the Navy. They will ascertain, as far as practicable, whether the recruit be subject to convulsions of any kind, or has received any contusion or wounds of the head which may produce occasional insanity. With any of these defects, the man will be rejected.

The surgeon also determined whether the applicant was protected from smallpox by vaccination or previous infection. If not, the recruit was vaccinated when transferred to a vessel, typically a receiving ship.[1]

The corresponding guidance document for Confederate surgeons was silent on the details of the examination and did not enumerate the conditions that should keep a man out of the navy.

12. Rendering Judgments

Since the CSN was chronically short of seamen, surgeons conducting examinations may have been relatively reluctant to declare men unfit for the service. In many cases, the medical officers assigned to rendezvous—Surgeons James Cornick, William F. Carrington, John T. Mason, and William B. Sinclair, for example—had long experience in the USN and may not have needed written criteria. In other instances, examining officers, such as Assistant Surgeons Luther R. Dickinson and William W. Graves, had no naval experience before entering the CSN. No person was to be accepted into the CSN unless the commander of the rendezvous and the medical officer there agreed on the applicant's fitness to serve. CSN rendezvous were established in Charleston, Macon, Mobile, New Orleans, Norfolk, Raleigh, Richmond, and Savannah.[2]

Robert R. Gibbes described in February 1861 his experiences at Charleston examining recruits from all parts of the world for the South Carolina navy. He was forced to declare a good number of them—many of whom were experienced sailors with chronic ailments—physically unfit for service. Gibbes, who would soon join the CSN as an assistant surgeon,

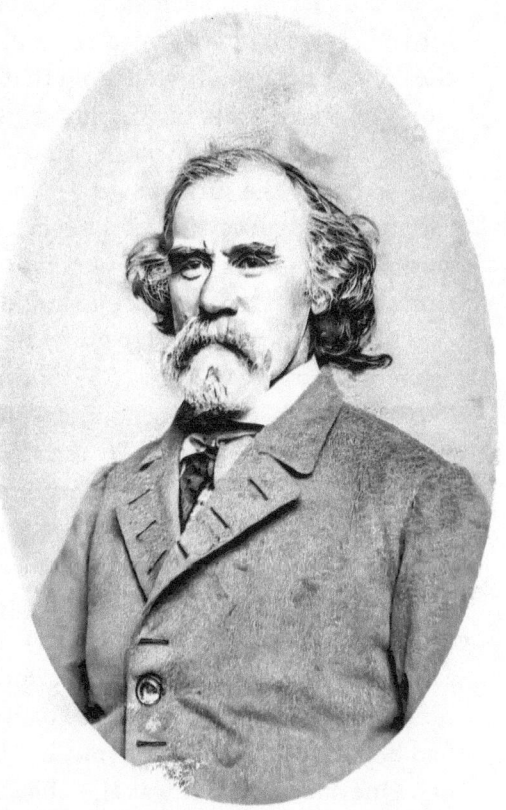

John T. Mason, who served as a CSN surgeon. Mason had been in the USN since 1837, resigned in May 1861, and spent much of his CSN time examining recruits. In this image, probably taken after the war, Mason appears to be wearing a CSN uniform coat without its military buttons (courtesy Jonathan O'Neal, M.D.).

The Confederate Navy Medical Corps

had little naval experience at the time, and it is unclear whether his examining criteria differed from those generally used once the war commenced. He added that his duties would have been more agreeable had all of the recruits bathed before he examined them.[3]

Applicants accepted into the navy were sent to a receiving ship for further processing, indoctrination, and training. There, a surgeon again determined the need for smallpox vaccination and administered the vaccine, if necessary. If that surgeon believed a recruit unfit for the service, he informed the ship's commander, who informed the commander of the station so that a survey—an official examination—could be ordered. The survey was conducted by at least three officers, at least one of whom had to be a medical officer and preferably senior to the surgeon at the rendezvous who had examined the recruit. If the survey found the recruit unfit, a report was sent to the station commander and the secretary of the navy for the latter's decision about whether the recruit should remain in the navy.[4]

Medical officers serving on receiving ships included Assistant Surgeons James O. Grant (CSS *Indian Chief*, Charleston), William W. Graves (CSS *Danube*, Mobile), William Sheppardson (CSS *Arctic*, Wilmington), and Samuel D. Drewry and Algernon S. Garnett (CSS *United States*, Norfolk). CSS *Sampson* was used as receiving ship at Savannah, but the CSN examining officer aboard—if any—has not been identified. In at least two cases, at least one of the physicians on a receiving ship was a civilian: Ralph Darby on CSS *St. Philip* (New Orleans) and G. Floyd Johnston on CSS *Dalman* (Mobile).[5]

The Confederacy's first conscription act in 1862 allowed the secretary of the navy to request the transfer to the CSN of seamen who had been drafted into the army, but that provision yielded few sailors. One such transfer was the object of Assistant Surgeon Thomas J. Charlton, Jr., in July 1862, when he was ordered to accompany Lieutenant Oscar F. Johnston, CSN, to the army's conscription center at Camp Randolph, near Calhoun, Georgia, to select "from the conscripts there the full complement of men for the floating battery *Georgia*." Charlton and Johnston were to return with the men to Savannah, but whether the mission was a success has not been determined.[6]

12. Rendering Judgments

Legislation of May 1, 1863, provided for the transfer of men from the army to the navy if those men so desired and the transfer was requested by the secretary of the navy. Subsequently, Assistant Surgeon William S. Stoakley, CSN, was ordered in June 1863 to assist Lieutenant Henry L. Graves of the Confederate States Marine Corps in obtaining recruits at the army conscript camp at Decatur, Georgia. Notwithstanding the results of that mission, which are unknown, the May 1, 1863, law was, according to Captain Sidney Smith Lee of the navy's Office of Orders and Detail, "disregarded entirely."[7]

On March 22, 1864, Adjutant and Inspector General Samuel Cooper of the War Department authorized the transfer of 1,200 soldiers to the navy. The Army of Tennessee was to relinquish 170 men, and Secretary Mallory dispatched Lieutenant W.W. Carnes and Assistant Surgeon Cincinnatus M. Parker to that army to make their selections and ensure that they were physically fit—this despite the fact that the soldiers, on entering the army, had supposedly been declared fit by an army surgeon. Carnes, satisfied with the transferees, a portion of whom were sent to Savannah under Parker's charge, reported that "as a general thing, the men are very good men; some of them are remarkably good men, and some very fine sailors. They are all reliable as far as patriotism and courage are concerned, for they have been well tried in the Army." By October 31, 1864, Cooper's order had resulted in 960 men from the armies east of the Mississippi being transferred to the navy. Other CSN surgeons involved in the transfers have not been identified.[8]

The assessment of army personnel treated by Passed Assistant Surgeon Robert R. Gibbes told a different story. During August 1864, Gibbes described the season as one of constant sickness and death, in which various sorts of fevers were afflicting the patients admitted to the Charleston Naval Hospital, where he was stationed. The ill came mainly from the receiving ship *Indian Chief* and from boat stations and consisted largely of army conscripts from North Carolina who had been assigned temporary naval duty. According to Gibbes, the patients seemed more animal than human, were feeble in constitution, and lacked moral or social principle. When acting in patients of such poor material, said Gibbes, bilious remittent fevers were usually fatal.[9]

Examination of Prospective Nonmedical Officers

CSN regulations stated that no person could "receive an original commission, warrant or appointment" in the navy or marines unless found physically qualified by one or more naval surgeons. Commissioned officers—including lieutenants and above, masters, midshipmen, surgeons, paymasters, and engineers—were nominated by the president and subject to approval by the Senate (or, before creation of a bicameral congress, by the Provisional Congress). Warrant officers included boatswains, gunners, carpenters, and sailmakers; they owed their status to the secretary of the navy. Appointed officers, named by senior officers, included secretary to a squadron commander, clerk to a commanding officer, and clerk to a paymaster. It appears that men who had been commissioned, warrant, or appointed officers in the USN, having already been examined before the war, needed no examination of physical fitness to become officers in the CSN. On the other hand, men enlisting as petty officers (including surgeons' stewards) or seamen, regardless of USN service, had to undergo a physical examination.[10]

Young men between 14 and 18 years of age applying for admission to the new Confederate States Navy Academy, based at Drewry's Bluff aboard CSS *Patrick Henry*, were to be examined for physical fitness by *Patrick Henry*'s surgeon and two other medical officers named by the secretary of the navy. Except for surveys for disability, described below, having three surgeons perform routine physical examinations was unique to the academy. The rationale was that a successful applicant had to be judged "qualified to discharge the arduous duties of an officer of the navy; both at the time of the examination, and probably, during the rest of his life, until age shall disable him." Academy regulations specified the medical conditions that would disqualify an applicant from admission. Medical officers with *Patrick Henry* during its service as the academy vessel included Assistant Surgeons William J. Addison and James G. Boxley. Other physicians involved in examining midshipmen included Surgeons Daniel B. Conrad, William D. Harrison, and Dinwiddie B. Phillips.

12. Rendering Judgments

One or more of *Patrick Henry*'s medical officers may also have examined newly released Confederate prisoners of war as they arrived for exchange from Harrison's Landing, which was downriver from Richmond and in Federal control. *Patrick Henry* received those former prisoners, a role that may have resulted in the vessel being called a receiving ship, albeit not in the usual sense.[11]

Examining for Disability

After the recruitment period, examining men for disability necessitated surveys that could involve multiple surgeons. Medical officers notified their commanding officer of men they thought might be physically unfit for service and should thus be surveyed. (An illness or injury that temporarily disqualified a man from duty did not merit a survey.) The commander, in turn, notified the senior officer in command, who ordered a survey to be conducted by at least one medical officer, and three if practicable. Thus, when Passed Assistant Surgeon Thomas J. Charlton, Jr., of CSS *Georgia* recommended on December 19, 1862, that Quartermaster J.J. Major be subjected to a survey, Lieutenant John Pembroke Jones, commanding *Georgia*, forwarded that recommendation to Flag Officer Josiah Tattnall of the Savannah Squadron. Tattnall then ordered Assistant Surgeon Theodosius Bartow Ford, Assistant Surgeon Robert J. Freeman, and Assistant Surgeon for the War Thomas Emory to conduct the survey; at least two of the three were from squadron vessels other than *Georgia*. (Assigning surveys to surgeons from other vessels was common, since surgeons recommending a survey were thought likely to have already formed an opinion on the matter.) The board found Major to be suffering from chronic rheumatism and unlikely to be fit for duty for several months and recommended on December 20, with Major's consent, that he be discharged from the navy. Major was discharged on December 25.[12]

In at least one circumstance, a sailor or marine might be examined by an army rather than a naval board. In February 1864, the Confederate Congress created the Invalid Corps, to be composed

The Confederate Navy Medical Corps

of military men who had been permanently disabled by wounds received or sickness contracted in the line of duty. Such persons would be discharged by a medical examining board and continue to receive their normal pay and emoluments until the end of the war or as long as they remained retired or discharged. The secretary of the army could detail an invalid to some duty that he was qualified to perform. A June 1864 amendment extended the provisions to personnel, including marines, who had not been specifically named in the original act, and provided that the secretary of the navy would make duty assignments for invalids of the navy or marines.[13]

When Corporal William Dunlop of the marines was referred to an army examining board for consideration for the Invalid Corps, the board initially considered the case out of its jurisdiction. That decision was overruled, since the legislation indicated that the applicant be examined by "one of the medical examining boards now established by law," without specifying that a marine or sailor had to be examined by a naval board. Dunlop was consequently seen by a board of three army surgeons. They found him permanently disabled because of the below-knee amputation of his right leg, a result of a battle wound sustained while serving on CSS *Atlanta*. The board retired Dunlop, which qualified him for the Invalid Corps.[14]

A board of survey looked into the health of at least one medical officer. In August 1863, Surgeon William F. McClenahan, who had recently been assigned as surgeon for CSS *Patrick Henry*, school ship for the Confederate Naval Academy, was found "unable owing to indisposition" to perform his duties. As the finding implied a disability that would not resolve quickly, McClenahan was ordered to the naval works at Charlotte, North Carolina, "to take charge of medical stores, and also to attend to the officers, and their families, on that Station." McClenahan, who had entered the USN in 1833 and was in his mid–50s when surveyed, was to inform the Office of Orders and Detail when he had recovered sufficiently to assume duty on shipboard. McClenahan's treatment seems quite accommodating, for if he had still been in the USN, he might well have been placed on the retired list, with removal from active service and reduction in pay.

12. Rendering Judgments

His unsuitability for service on *Patrick Henry* was consistent with his being omitted the next year from the PNCS.[15]

Other Examinations

Surveys could also be performed on supplies thought to be defective. They were to be performed by at least two commissioned officers "of a rank proportioned to the importance of the survey to be held." When performed on a ship, the surveying officers were to be selected, if possible, from another vessel. Since no other CSN vessels were nearby, Passed Assistant Surgeons Joseph D. Grafton, Jr., and Frederic Garretson participated with six other officers, all among CSS *Florida*'s complement, in examining a load of Cardiff coal received in Havana and in questioning the ship's engineers. While off the Cuban coast, the board concluded that the coal, "though admirable in appearance," did not "make a lively fire" and would not provide the cruiser with the necessary speed. Enough should be thrown overboard, suggested the board, to allow access to better coal previously received at Mobile, which should be used to take *Florida* to England, where better coal could be obtained to replace the Cardiff coal. Although not all of the officers on the board were chosen because of their knowledge of coal or engines, they were expected to interview crewmembers, such as engineers, who had such expertise.[16]

Although fleet surgeons supervised their squadrons' medical officers, specifics about fleet surgeons conducting inspections did not appear in naval regulations. Flag officers, however, were required by regulations to order "frequent inspections of hospitals and hospital ships" and to conduct inspections of squadron vessels quarterly, if practicable, and at other times as needed. Thus, Flag Officer John K. Mitchell of the James River Squadron, ordered seven officers in January 1865 to conduct the quarterly inspection of the squadron. The group included the lieutenant of the flagship (*Virginia II*), Fleet Surgeon William D. Harrison, a passed midshipman, a marine lieutenant, and three engineers.[17]

Mitchell also directed six medical officers from four different vessels of the James River Squadron—Fleet Surgeon William D. Harrison, Surgeon Henry W.M. Washington, and Assistant Surgeons James W. Belvin, Henry G. Land, John Leyburn, and James E. Moyler—to report their opinion of the "substance now issued as coffee" complained of by Assistant Surgeon Pike Brown of CSS *Richmond*. (Among substances that were "brevetted coffee" in the squadron were "hot water colored with chicory or burnt grains of corn" and "a decoction of sweet potatoes or beans.") Unfortunately, the group's report has not been found. It may not have been considered a formal survey, which was to be reported in triplicate, since Mitchell asked for the report in duplicate only.[18]

Another investigation that was probably not a formal survey was conducted by Surgeons William B. Sinclair, James F. Harrison, and William F. Carrington. OMS chief Spotswood asked the three to investigate the causes of illness in the James River Squadron. They concluded that the contributing factors were the presence of malaria where the vessels were anchored, the "heated atmosphere of the ironclads," a lack of proper exercise, and a deficiency of vegetables and fruit. They suggested anchoring the fleet in a healthier place, if possible, providing wind sails or other sources of ventilation, allowing crews to exercise on shore, increasing the amounts of vegetables and fruit, and using awnings. The board also recommended that the whiskey ration be given with hot coffee early each morning.[19]

Courts

Naval surgeons could serve in courts of inquiry and courts-martial. In June 1864, for example, Surgeon James W.B. Greenhow served as judge advocate for the court of inquiry that investigated the loss of CSS *Raleigh* near Wilmington. The court found no negligence or inattention on the part of anyone aboard.[20]

In another instance, Surgeons William B. Sinclair and James F. Harrison were among nine naval officers composing the court-martial of Surgeon Algernon S. Garnett. (USN regulations, adopted by the CSN, directed that a court of inquiry or court-martial trying

12. Rendering Judgments

a medical officer, paymaster, or engineer should have at least one officer of the same corps on the court.) In November 1862, Garnett was tried on two charges. The first, "scandalous conduct, or conduct unbecoming an officer and gentleman," asserted that Garnett had used improper language toward marine lieutenant James F. Claiborne, was drunk or sufficiently under the influence of liquor to attract attention, and assaulted and struck marine captain Alfred C. Van Benthuysen. The incidents allegedly occurred on October 2, 1862, during a party or picnic at Drewry's Bluff at which ladies and gentlemen were present. The second charge was that Garnett had quarreled with and threatened to attack Claiborne. The specification alleged that Garnett uttered of Claiborne, "I will slap his face" and sought him out for that purpose. The court found that the specification of the first charge had not been proved and that Garnett was not guilty of the first charge. The specification of the second charge, said the court, had been proved, but Garnett was not guilty of the second charge. The final verdict was that Garnett was honorably acquitted of both charges.[21]

Secretary Mallory thought the verdict was improper and directed the court to reconsider its findings. After the court returned with the same findings, Mallory was forced, "under the existing laws and usage of the service ... to approve the proceedings and acquiesce in the finding and sentence of the court." Mallory, however, persisted in his opinion of the verdict and publicized his "strong disapproval" and "emphatic rebuke" of the court's decision in a general order published repeatedly in Richmond newspapers in January 1863. Some newspapers condemned Mallory for his behavior. The *Richmond Whig*, for example, said that Garnett's altercation was "a private affair which might befall any gentleman" and faulted Mallory, first, for bringing it to the public arena by convening a court-martial and, second, for failing to quietly abide by the court's initial decision. On the other hand, a Charlotte newspaper opined that acquittal was expected because "of course ... such bodies scarcely ever convict an officer" and that Mallory was right to speak up if he thought the court had failed in its duty. The court's findings may have been influenced by the fact that its president was Commodore George N.

Hollins, who had helped in 1861 to seize the steamer *St. Nicholas* and was aided by Garnett when that ship then captured three prize vessels. Incidents probably related to the court's findings included Garnett being detached from Drewry's Bluff in December 1862 and Lieutenant Claiborne being dismissed from the marine corps on January 14, 1863.[22]

In a separate trial in October 1862, Captain Van Benthuysen was convicted of at least one charge for his part in the altercation with Garnett and sentenced to be dismissed from the service. Secretary Mallory recommended mitigation of the sentence, and President Jefferson Davis shortened it to suspension from rank and command for four months.[23]

Secretary Mallory's public condemnation of Garnett's acquittal—and indirectly of Surgeon Garnett himself and the members of his court-martial—prompted the introduction of a bill that would prohibit the secretary of the navy from commenting on the acquittal of the accused party at a naval court-martial, other than endorsing the written court proceedings as "approved" or "sanctioned" for his agreement or disagreement, respectively, with the court's decision. Although the bill was passed by the Confederate Senate, it was tabled by the House of Representatives.[24]

Medical officers were probably members of the court-martial of another fellow physician, Assistant Surgeon John C. Harrison. Nothing has been found regarding the charges against Harrison or the court's findings, but his trial occurred in Richmond in June 1863, with Captain Sidney Smith Lee as presiding officer, Andrew H. Sands as judge advocate, and Commander Robert B. Pegram as a witness. By September 1863, Harrison had been assigned to CSS *Selma* of the Mobile Squadron.[25]

* * *

The expertise of CSN medical officers was called upon in making judgments about the physical fitness of recruits and officer candidates. When the physical ability of naval or marine personnel to perform their duties was called into question, surgeons were tasked with examining the men in question and determining whether to

12. Rendering Judgments

recommend their discharge from the service. Panels that included medical officers were also assembled to inquire into the quality of supplies and into conditions affecting the health of naval personnel. Finally, medical officers could be assigned as members of courts of inquiry and courts-martial and were probably most likely to be selected when a fellow medical officer was the subject of the proceeding. Assignments were probably based on surgeons' perceived medical expertise and overall objectivity.

– 13 –

Sundry Activities

Confederate naval medical officers were usually assigned to vessels, hospitals, recruiting stations, or navy yards. At times, however, they could find themselves with postings—or with ad hoc duties—that still called on their skills and judgment but might nevertheless be considered outside their usual responsibilities.

Expeditions and Raids

Naval surgeons sometimes participated in expeditions or raids, where their skills in treating wounds might be needed. Perhaps the first such episode involved the passenger steamer *St. Nicholas*, which ran regularly between Baltimore and Washington, D.C. In late July 1861, Confederates posing as passengers and led by Colonel Richard Thomas of the Maryland Zouaves and Captain George N. Hollins, CSN, seized the vessel near Point Lookout, Maryland. They proceeded to the Coan River Landing on the Virginia side of the Potomac River, where a group of Confederate soldiers and sailors came aboard to assist; they included Algernon S. Garnett, who had just received his commission as assistant surgeon, CSN, and was awaiting an assignment. With its new crew, *St. Nicholas* quickly captured three prize vessels on the Chesapeake Bay before sailing up the Rappahannock to Fredericksburg, where *St. Nicholas* was purchased by the Confederate government.[1]

Garnett just happened to be handy when *St. Nicholas* took on men to help in its mission, but including CSN surgeons on expeditions and raids was typically more deliberate. It was not unusual at the time for medical officers to be included in boarding parties,

13. Sundry Activities

landing operations, or expeditions. Among the supplies routinely carried by a ship's boat during such excursions were tourniquets, bandages, medicines, and surgical implements.[2]

In January 1864, Surgeon Daniel B. Conrad, then serving at Drewry's Bluff, was ordered to report to North Carolina as a member of a party to undertake an as-yet undisclosed operation. The mission was to seize a USN gunboat, and the target ended up being USS *Underwriter*, anchored off the coast of New Bern, North Carolina, which the party seized on February 2. The raiders, consisting of about 120 men in 10 boats, approached the vessel at night, boarded it, and captured it after brief fighting. Conrad watched the hand-to-hand struggle from *Underwriter*'s wheelhouse, having "nothing to do as yet" until his comrades shouted that *Underwriter* was theirs. Conrad then leaped to the deck, slipped on blood, fell, and was nearly shot by a fellow CSN officer, who then took the surgeon to see a fallen comrade. While examining the man, remembered Conrad, "I felt my hand slip down between his ears, and to my horror, discovered that his head had been cleft in two by a boarding sword in the hands of some giant of the forecastle." Conrad ordered that the bodies of the killed be gathered and found several wounded men below in the ward room. Although the party intended to use *Underwriter* to attack other Federal vessels, the ship could not be quickly freed from its mooring, and it was taking fire from a Federal fort, whose occupants had learned of *Underwriter*'s capture. The dead and wounded were placed in the boats, which departed for shore after officers of the raiding part set *Underwriter* ablaze. "I boarded boat after boat in my capacity of surgeon," said Conrad, "attending to the requirements of those who demanded immediate aid." Among the prisoners in the boats were officers and men whom Conrad recognized from his USN service.[3]

In June 1864, Assistant Surgeons C. Wesley Thomas and William C. Jones were members of a 132-man party in seven boats that captured the Federal gunboat *Water Witch*, part of the blockading fleet off the coast of Georgia. Before the capture, Thomas participated in a reconnoitering expedition and was left on an island with two other men to watch their target; they were picked up later when

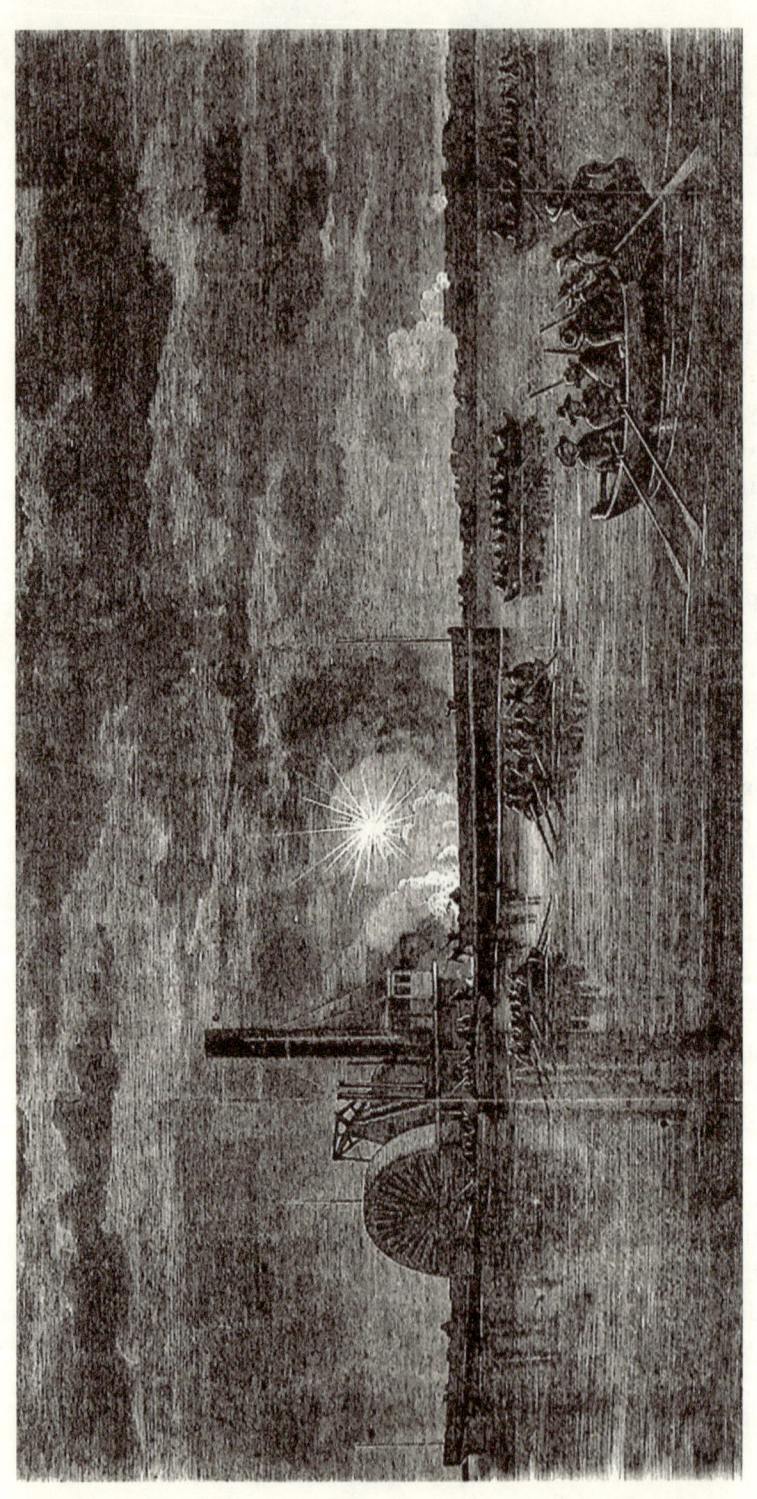

Boats manned by CSN personnel, including Surgeon Daniel B. Conrad, during a night raid on USS *Underwriter*, February 2, 1864, near New Bern, North Carolina. Conrad boarded *Underwriter* and later treated both CSN and USN wounded (*Frank Leslie's Illustrated Newspaper*, Jan. 28, 1864).

13. Sundry Activities

the entire party approached *Water Witch*. Casualties resulting from the boarding and subsequent fighting totaled 16 among the Federals (one killed, 13 wounded, two missing) and a larger number among the Confederates (six to eight killed outright, two mortally wounded, and 15–20 wounded less seriously). Acting Assistant Surgeon W.H. Pierson, USN, of *Water Witch* treated his shipmates in various parts of the vessel and reported having Thomas's assistance. Thomas was mentioned by Flag Officer William W. Hunter, CSN, as one of the raiders who "markedly distinguished themselves."[4]

A medical officer, Assistant Surgeon William Sheppardson, was included in a party of 82 officers and men in four boats that captured two Federal gunboats, *Satellite* and *Reliance*, at the mouth of the Rappahannock River in August 1863. During that exploit, three Confederate raiders were wounded; Federal losses were two killed and four wounded. The raid's commander, Lieutenant John Taylor Wood, CSN, reported that all officers and men, including Sheppardson, "did their duty."[5]

Assistant Surgeon William S. Stoakley was part of two small reconnaissance missions in December 1864 on the Savannah River. During the second trip, the party came under rifle fire but escaped unharmed. A final example involved the aforementioned Assistant Surgeon Sheppardson, who was among 22 men, mostly from the CSN, who entered Canada in late 1863 intending to capture USS *Michigan*, the only Federal war vessel sailing the Great Lakes, and free the Confederate prisoners held at Johnson's Island, in Sandusky Bay near the Ohio shore. The expedition was foiled when a Canadian man thought to be sympathetic to the Southerners' cause informed an official of the plot, which resulted in U.S. secretary of war Edwin Stanton notifying mayors of cities on the lakes to guard against a Confederate raid and sending reinforcements to Johnson's Island. The raiders abandoned their plan and left Canada without incident.[6]

Including surgeons on dangerous expeditions provided for medical care and probably satisfied the medical officers' desire for adventure or took advantage of their leadership abilities. The same motives probably applied when the Confederate cruiser *Florida* captured the bark *Lapwing* in the mid–Atlantic on March 28, 1863, and transferred to that vessel a howitzer and 18 crewmembers, including Passed Assistant Surgeon Joseph D. Grafton, Jr., *Lapwing* then commenced its own hunt for prize vessels, and on May 3, 1863, Grafton transferred back to CSS *Florida* when both vessels met off the coast of Brazil. Grafton died on May 29 when a boat he and shipmates took to shore overturned.[7]

Other Assignments

In at least one instance, a CSN surgeon was given a mission evidently unrelated to his medical background. Assistant Surgeon George A. Foote was on the ironclad ram *Albemarle* on October 27, 1864, when that vessel was moored at Plymouth, North Carolina, on the Roanoke River, about eight miles from Albemarle Sound. On that night, a launch captained by Lieutenant William B. Cushing, USN, approached *Albemarle* under fire, and Cushing detonated a torpedo (mine) against the ram's hull and sank it. The loss of *Albemarle* left the troops at Plymouth in danger because of nearby Union forces, so the Confederate army's district commander, Brigadier General Laurence S. Baker, ordered Foote "to take command there and extricate the garrison from their perilous position." The evacuation occurred without loss of a single man, and Foote was commended for his skill and gallantry. According to naval regulations, staff officers, such as surgeons, had "authority to exercise command ... in matters relating to duties in their own corps, but not in any other corps" except when that authority was "specially extended." General Baker's order evidently constituted such specially extended authority.[8]

After the battle between CSS *Virginia* and USS *Monitor* in March 1862, Flag Officer Franklin Buchanan, CSN, recovering from a wound at the Confederate army (formerly naval) hospital at Norfolk, sent *Virginia*'s surgeon, Dinwiddie B. Phillips, to Richmond with an urgent dispatch for Secretary Mallory, to be delivered in person. Phillips handed the dispatch to Mallory and drew his attention to Buchanan's suggestion that the James River be obstructed against Union vessels. According to Phillips, Mallory "threw the paper

13. Sundry Activities

carelessly aside, without reading a page." Notwithstanding the snub, Buchanan's confidence in Phillips was demonstrated, and when the surgeon returned to Norfolk, he found *Virginia* "with steam up and only awaiting my arrival before revisiting the [Hampton] Roads."[9]

While aboard CSS *Lady Davis*, Assistant Surgeon Robert R. Gibbes was ordered ashore to procure some axes that were needed immediately. Another task assigned to Gibbes while assigned to that vessel—which was stationed near Charleston, where no paymaster was present at the time—was to take a train to Savannah to collect the officers' pay from the paymaster there.[10]

After Lieutenant General Leonidas Polk, Episcopal Bishop of the Diocese of Louisiana, was killed at Pine Mountain, Georgia, on June 18, 1864, Bishop Stephen Elliott of the Diocese of Georgia, asked that naval officers of the Savannah Station attend Polk's funeral in Augusta. Captain Josiah Tatnall, commandant of the CSN's Savannah Station thus ordered Surgeon Richard W. Jeffery of the Savannah Naval Hospital, to attend the obsequies.[11]

Shore Assignments at War's End

Shortly before the evacuation of Richmond began on April 2, 1865, Rear Admiral Raphael Semmes, commanding the James River Squadron, was ordered by Secretary Mallory to destroy his ships and gather his forces in an attempt to join up with General Robert E. Lee, who was withdrawing toward Danville, Virginia. After destroying the vessels, Semmes and his men found two train engines and cars remaining in Richmond—many government officials had already fled by rail—and made their way to Danville, where they found President Jefferson Davis and Secretary Mallory. It was quickly decided that Semmes's command would be formed into a brigade of artillery, with Semmes assuming the grade of army brigadier general, and assigned to the defenses around Danville, the new seat of the Confederate government. Semmes divided his command of about 400 men into two regiments and assigned army grades to their officers. Semmes's Naval Brigade, as it came to be called, was occupying trenches near

Danville when informed of General Lee's surrender of the Army of Northern Virginia on April 9 at Appomattox Court House. Semmes then received orders from General Joseph E. Johnston to proceed to Greensboro, North Carolina, where the brigade was eventually paroled on May 1 as part of the Confederate Army of Tennessee. By then, Semmes's command, which had dwindled because of desertions, numbered about 250 men.[12]

Naval medical officers in Semmes's Brigade included Surgeon William D. Harrison, fleet surgeon of the James River Squadron, now army major and surgeon on the brigade's general staff; Assistant Surgeons John P. Lipscomb and James O. Grant, now surgeon and assistant surgeon, respectively, of the first regiment; and Assistant Surgeons Henry B. Melvin and Howell A. Venable, now surgeon and assistant surgeon, respectively, of the second regiment. Naval medical officers "attached to Brigade for special services" included Assistant Surgeons James W. Belvin, James E. Moyler, C. Wesley Thomas, Frederick Peck, James G. Boxley, Edmund K. Goldsborough, William D. Sale, and George C. Daniel. Belvin, Moyler, and Thomas had been given army grades of captain, first lieutenant, and second lieutenant, respectively, but grades were not recorded for the remaining CSN assistant surgeons.[13]

Captain John R. Tucker, CSN, was in command at Drewry's Bluff when Richmond was evacuated but received neither notification about the evacuation nor orders about what to do with his troops, many of whom had recently served at the naval stations and squadrons at Charleston and Wilmington. Tucker joined the rear guard of the Confederate army as part of Major General George Washington Custis Lee's division of Lieutenant General Richard S. Ewell's corps of the Army of Northern Virginia. Tucker's Brigade (or Battalion) fought stubbornly at the April 6, 1865, Battle of Sailor's (Sayler's) Creek and surrendered. Among the 300 or so men of Tucker's Brigade captured at the battle, none (according to one source) were CSN medical officers. However, Surgeon Francis L. Galt and Assistant Surgeons George N. Halstead and Gustave E. Sussdorff—reported to have been part of the brigade—were paroled at Appomattox Court House on April 9, probably after evading capture at Sailor's Creek.[14]

13. Sundry Activities

* * *

Miscellaneous duties assigned to medical officers included accompanying raiding parties and commanding army personnel. At the end of the war, some surgeons, relieved of their naval responsibilities, cooperated with elements of the army. Such ad hoc assignments seemed to take advantage of medical officers' professional and leadership qualities.

– 14 –

End and Aftermath of the War

The fire that consumed much of Richmond on April 3, 1865—initially set by fleeing Confederate troops to destroy bridges and tobacco warehouses—claimed various government buildings. Among them was the Virginia Mechanics Institute, which had housed War and Navy Department offices, including the OMS. Union troops began occupying Richmond the same day. A New York newspaper correspondent, writing on April 4, described the Mechanics Institute, formerly "a handsome, brick building," as being "now in smoking ruins." It is unclear whether the Richmond Naval Hospital, which was adjacent to or within the fire zone, survived the blaze. Historian Rebecca Barbour Calcutt indicates that Naval Hospital patients were transferred to Richmond's Winder Hospital, which had been used by the Confederate army, on April 8, 1865. If true, patients could have been evacuated from the Naval Hospital during the fire, moved back to that facility when the danger was over, and then transferred to Winder. According to a Northern reporter, all Confederate patients remaining in Richmond hospitals were moved by April 10 to Jackson Hospital, a facility formerly operated by the Confederate army and located in Richmond's western suburbs.[1]

When Richmond was evacuated, OMS chief Spotswood was elsewhere on a leave of absence, and Surgeon James F. Harrison was probably acting in his stead. Harrison's parole in Richmond on April 28, 1865, suggests that he remained in the city while President Jefferson Davis, the president's cabinet, and various other government officials, including Secretary Mallory, fled Richmond by rail, on their way to Danville, Virginia. Surgeon General Samuel Preston

14. End and Aftermath of the War

Moore of the army also appears to have escaped Richmond at about the same time, but no evidence has been found that any CSN medical officer stationed at the capital—as opposed to serving with the James River Squadron or at Drewry's Bluff—left the city on April 2 or 3. Also surrendering in Richmond were Assistant Surgeons John DeBree, Jr., William Mason Turner, and John H. Tucker on April 3, and Surgeon William F. Patton on April 6. Medical officers paroled shortly after the war's end in Richmond—their surrender dates are not available—included Surgeons Richard W. Jeffery and William M. Page and Assistant Surgeons Richard C. Bowles, William W. Coggin, and Thomas J. Wheeden. One or more of these paroled officers may have been serving at the Naval Hospital or the OMS.[2]

Thirteen medical officers serving with the James River Squadron constituted part of Semmes's Naval Brigade and were paroled at Greensboro, North Carolina, on May 1. Another 12 medical officers were among the men paroled at Nanna Hubba Bluff on the Tombigbee River, Alabama. Other locales where naval surgeons are known to have been paroled include Selma, Alabama; Tallahassee, Florida; Augusta and Macon, Georgia; Jackson, Mississippi; and Appomattox Court House, Dover Mines, and Lynchburg, Virginia.[3]

Surgeon Spotswood was paroled on April 21, 1865, at an undetermined location and submitted written pleas for pardon, from Pensacola, on June 28 and August 23, 1865. The requests were required because amnesty was not granted automatically to men who had resigned U.S. military commissions to aid the rebellion. Not having received the desired response, Spotswood applied again in February 1867, stating that only with a pardon could he dispose of "a few acres of pine wood land ... all of which would not sell for five hundred dollars," a sum that was nevertheless needed to keep his family from starving. The application was supported by William Marvin, former provisional governor of Florida, who represented Spotswood as poverty-stricken. U.S. Attorney General Henry Stanbery recommended a pardon, which was granted on June 8, 1867. The reason behind the delay has not been determined, but former army surgeon general Moore also had to wait—until December 1, 1866—for his pardon. The delay in Moore's case was probably related to his having been implicated, although never formally accused or tried, in the mistreatment of prisoners of war.⁴

Former Passed Assistant Surgeon Robert R. Gibbes, after ending his medical services in Charlotte, North Carolina, on April 14, 1865, visited Columbia, South Carolina, in June and was not allowed to leave without a parole. He went to the Federal headquarters there and refused to sign a loyalty oath but managed nonetheless to secure a parole. Declining the oath, said Gibbes, resulted in his being registered as an enemy of the United States, a designation he seemed to relish.⁵

Most former CSN surgeons appear to have entered civilian medical practice soon after the war, mostly in Southern states. Among the exceptions were Bennett W. Green, who was a passed assistant surgeon on the armored ram *Stonewall*, a French-built vessel that arrived at Nassau after the war's end and proceeded to Havana, where it was sold to pay the crew. Green declared that he "would not live in the same country with the Yankees," traveled to Liverpool, settled in Argentina, and eventually returned to his native Virginia in the 1880s. Another excep-

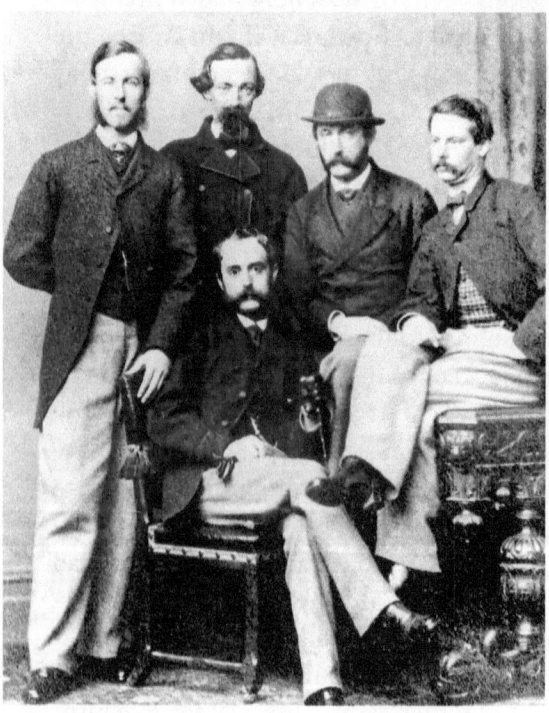

Autumn 1865 photograph of former CSN officers, including (with former grade) Assistant Surgeon Edwin G. Booth (seated, center) and, from left, Acting Master Irvine S. Bulloch, Passed Assistant Surgeon Bennett W. Green, First Lieutenant William H. Murdaugh, and Passed Assistant Surgeon Charles E. Lining. Green and Lining resided in Argentina after the war before returning to the United States (NHHC, image NH 59499).

14. End and Aftermath of the War

tion was Charles E. Lining, a passed assistant surgeon on the commerce-raider *Shenandoah*, which ended its cruise at Liverpool some six months after the war ended. Lining, too, settled in Argentina before he returned to the United States in 1874, locating at Evansville, Indiana, and then at Paducah, Kentucky.[6]

Former Assistant Surgeon Stephen S. Herrick wrote numerous articles for medical journals after the war, whereas the postwar writings of former Surgeons Daniel B. Conrad and Dinwiddie B. Phillips emphasized nonmedical aspects of their Civil War experiences. Former Assistant Surgeon Edwin G. Booth wrote to the U.S. Navy Department to point out an error in its 1898 summary of his CSN service; he had actually served on CSS *Selma* rather than CSS *Tuscaloosa*. Former Surgeon Francis L. Galt also wanted to set the record straight when he disputed the accuracy of an 1886 story in *Century Magazine* about life on CSS *Alabama*, on which he served. The magazine editors later acknowledged being duped by the article's author, who had not served on *Alabama* as previously claimed, and consequently having doubts about the story's credibility. Former Passed Assistant Surgeon Frederic Garretson published articles on both medical and nonmedical topics.[7]

Details about the postwar life of William A.W. Spotswood are sketchy. He was appointed as quarantine physician at Pensacola in 1866, 1868, and 1878. In 1874, he was named chairman of the Committee on Naval Service of the Association of Medical Officers of the Late Confederate Army and Navy, but details about that service have not been found. In 1884, Spotswood's wife, the former Mary Eastin, died in Mobile. In 1889, Spotswood was reported to be living at Point Clear, Baldwin County, Alabama. Spotswood died on September 7, 1891, at the Providence Infirmary in Mobile. He is not known to have left any written account of his CSN service.[8]

Conclusion

A few days after Union troops marched into a burning Richmond in April 1865, a Northern reporter stated that attempts to check the fire had "seemed as impotent as if they had been directed against Vesuvius." Although the blaze had spread quickly on its own, the correspondent speculated that the War and Quartermaster Department headquarters, where the OMS and other Navy Department offices were also located, "may have been fired independently, as load on loads of papers were hauled out into the street and burned on Sunday [April 2]." Indeed, Secretary of the Navy Mallory said that most Navy Department records were destroyed during and shortly after evacuation of the capital. Other official documents were apparently transported to the Charlotte Navy Yard and destroyed there.[1]

The loss and dispersal of Confederate records at the end of the Civil War have made it difficult to form a complete picture of how the CSN's medical department operated. Particularly useful would have been documents amassed and tabulated by the OMS in Richmond. A complete set of letters sent and received by the OMS, for example, would have been extremely helpful, as would summary statistics on the number and medical problems of patients treated. The lack of CSN data in the massive *Medical and Surgical History of the War of the Rebellion* is conspicuous and makes it difficult for researchers to compare medical conditions and care between the Union and Confederate navies or between the Confederate army and navy. A wartime diary or journal kept by OMS chief Spotswood or one of his assistants might have provided some context to help explain why certain actions were taken. Except for three reports from Spotswood to Secretary Mallory, there is little to indicate Spotswood's reasoning, management style, or personality.[2]

Conclusion

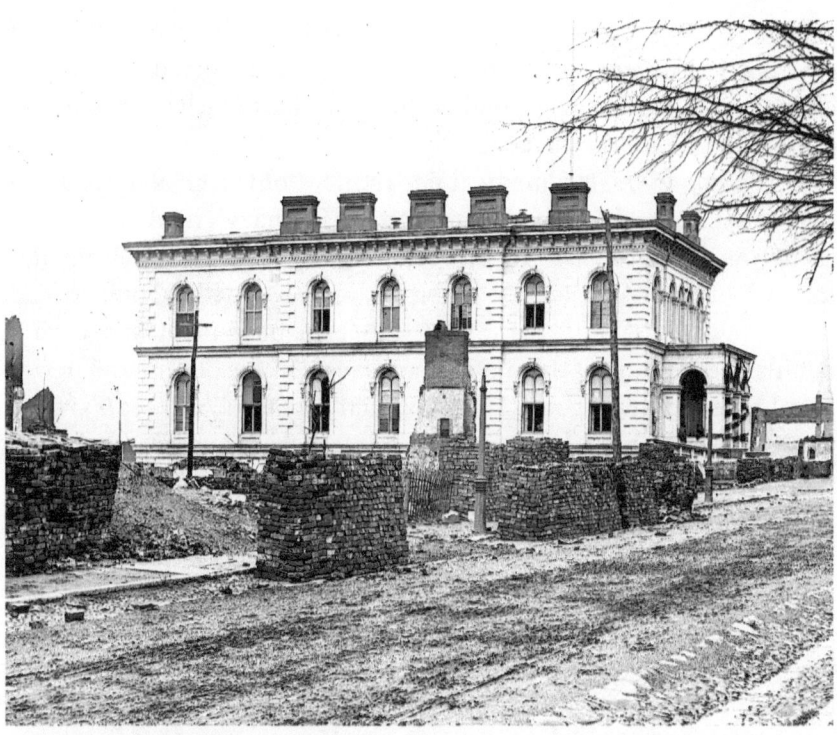

The Custom House (also called the Treasury Building) in Richmond shortly after fire consumed most of the surrounding structures in April 1865. This building housed the Confederate War and Navy Departments for about a month in 1861 before they moved to the building of the Virginia Mechanics Institute (also destroyed), less than a block away beyond the right edge of the photograph (Library of Congress, control no. 2018666786).

Topics remain about which almost nothing is known. How involved, for example, was the OMS in seeking new legislation to bolster the number of medical officers and enhance their standing within the navy? How did political considerations affect the scope and types of services that the naval medical department was able to provide? How well did Surgeon Spotswood handle such political complications? Exactly how many land-based naval hospitals existed, where were they, and how were they staffed? How were medical services managed west of the Mississippi River, especially after that region was effectively isolated when control of the river was seized by the Union? What steps did the OMS take to keep its medical officers

183

Conclusion

informed about treating ailments they were likely to see? To what extent did the navy provide dental and other specialized care? What changes occurred near the end of the war, a period whose documentation is particularly sketchy?

In some ways, the medical department of the CSN is easier to study than that of the Confederate army. The navy's medical department was a much smaller organization having to treat a much smaller number of men. A large proportion of the CSN's medical officers had served in the USN and all, or nearly all, have been identified, even if details about many of them remain elusive. On the other hand, fewer naval than army surgeons left unofficial accounts of their wartime experiences, so it is difficult to get a feel for what naval medical practice was like.

The level of military and medical competence in naval surgeons was probably as high as could be reasonably expected. More than a third had been medical officers in the USN, and many others had been full or assistant surgeons in the Confederate army. All, or nearly all, physicians entering the CSN as medical officers had passed an examination by a board of USN or CSN surgeons. Spotswood seemed pleasantly surprised at the performance of his new assistant surgeons, reporting them to be, as a group, efficient and "evincing a competency not to be expected from inexperienced young men, just commencing their professional career."[3] There did seem to be discrepancies between the number of medical officers available or desired by the OMS and the assignments available to them. Early in the war, for example, a substantial number of CSN surgeons were assigned duty with the army, not only because the army needed them but because not enough naval postings existed for them. Later in the war, OMS chief Spotswood regularly asked that more slots for full surgeons be allowed. The large number of civilian physicians employed by the CSN implies frequent mismatches between local needs and the number and distribution of medical officers. The formation of the PNCS presented an opportunity to promote any number of passed assistant surgeons—a move that would have answered Spotswood's appeals for more full surgeons—yet no such promotions occurred.

Conclusion

As was the case in the USN, CSN surgeons sought higher status—as expressed by grade and pay—in relation to other naval and army officers. Legislative attempts to satisfy such aspirations were unsuccessful, possibly because they were considered to be relatively unimportant by Confederate lawmakers.

While the prewar USN had Home, Mediterranean, Pacific, Brazil, Africa, and East India Squadrons, most CSN vessels patrolled home waters. Thus, although CSN crewmembers were fairly unlikely to suffer from scurvy as long as they could procure fresh fruit and vegetables from the mainland, they were at high risk of contracting malaria when stationed in coastal areas where mosquitoes thrived. Although navy-wide statistics showing the comparative frequencies of diagnoses in the CSN are unavailable, malaria was certainly the health concern that most compromised the navy's fighting efficiency.

Unlike their army counterparts, CSN surgeons appear not to have had particular worries about medical evacuation unless they were involved in land battles. Sick or wounded men on vessels were first treated aboard and then transferred, if needed, to a floating or land-based hospital. Should naval hospitals be inadequate for the number of patients, naval surgeons could call on army or civilian hospitals for assistance.

Union naval prisoners were initially treated, if necessary, by CSN surgeons—sometimes with assistance from USN surgeons—and then turned over to the Confederate army. Thus, CSN surgeons were not tasked, as some of their army brethren were, with providing medical care in filthy and overcrowded prisons and escaped subsequent charges of abuse and neglect. Practices regarding the imprisonment of medical officers varied during the war such that some CSN surgeons taken prisoner were quickly released or exchanged, while others remained incarcerated for extended periods.

Unless newly captured USN hospitals were available for use, as was the case at Pensacola and Norfolk, the CSN tended to send men needing prolonged or definitive treatment to army or civilian hospitals instead of or before establishing their own. Such a strategy seems reasonable in light of the time needed to form shore facilities that were large enough to employ the number of sailors and

Conclusion

marines needed to justify a hospital. There is no evidence that parts of or entire naval hospitals became specialized—for the treatment of smallpox, for example—as army hospitals did. The medical officers assigned to shore establishments that were too small for a naval hospital probably set up dispensaries to handle minor ailments and used civilian hospitals or private physicians to treat more serious cases.

It seems unlikely that the OMS, as opposed to the Confederate army medical department, was heavily pressured by politicians to devote specific resources, such as hospitals, to military personnel from their state. The navy, after all, did not have regiments of men from the various Southern states, and its enlisted men were largely foreign-born. The CSN's hospital system was simply too small—in the number of facilities and patients—to allow the establishment of state-specific hospitals. Southern newspapers and congressional records reveal little if any publicly expressed dissatisfaction with the medical care provided by the CSN. Confederate army surgeons were often criticized by soldiers, civilians, and lawmakers for being incompetent or neglectful, with many complaints stemming from sick or injured men suffering delays in evacuation and treatment. One explanation for the difference is that a sailor injured on a vessel of war (on which a surgeon was present) "has not to fear being left behind" and "has not to suffer long hours of agony whilst waiting for help to reach him." Naval surgeons were also less likely than their army counterparts to be suddenly overwhelmed with huge numbers of wounded men.[4]

When not assigned traditional duty afloat in home waters or at hospitals, navy yards, or naval stations, medical officers often found themselves posted to shore batteries manned by sailors and marines. Some were sent to Europe to serve on commerce raiders. Medical officers occasionally took part in expeditions, such as daring and stealthy raids meant to capture unsuspecting enemy vessels. The judgment of medical officers was needed not only in the examination of recruits, officer candidates, and naval personnel thought to be disabled, it was often sought for courts of inquiry, courts-martial, and surveys of naval supplies thought to be faulty.

Although OMS chief Spotswood intended Richmond to be the

Conclusion

hub through which medical supplies were distributed to vessels and naval stations, large amounts of goods were purchased by medical officers in their own localities. It is not clear why regional medical purveying depots were not established at least at Charleston and Wilmington, the ports most frequently visited by blockade-runners. There is some evidence that medication shortages contributed to the use of nonstandard drugs, but it appears that the CSN did not take aggressive steps, as the army did, to make more use of medicines made from indigenous plants. It is doubtful that the OMS's purveying department was as successful in stocking vessels and stations with supplies as Spotswood indicated in his reports to Mallory.

What, then, can be said about the CSN's medical department? Its service, provided by a carefully assembled staff, was indispensable and from all indications—and in light of its many obstacles—its performance appears to have been quite creditable. Medical officers spent much time treating disease, particularly malaria, which was prevalent in Southern coastal areas, where most Confederate sailors and marines were stationed. There is no question that illness, at times, markedly reduced manpower. The vessels in the Mobile Squadron, during the summer of 1863, were about half-manned because of sickness, death, disability-related discharge, and desertion. A year later, one third of the men in the James River Squadron and the related batteries were sick. It is highly likely that the efforts of medical officers, many of whom were taken ill themselves, not only reduced suffering but prevented the manpower crises from becoming even worse. Beneficial actions of surgeons may have extended beyond actual medical care to advising commanders about locations where the risk of disease was lower.[5]

Surgeons were often praised by commanding officers for their coolness and leadership in battle, whether afloat or ashore. That surgeons faced the same hazards as other naval personnel is illustrated by the fact that at least 16 medical officers—out of about 100 who were commissioned and actually served—were taken prisoner while serving on vessels or at shore batteries. Six commissioned and one civilian medical officer died during the war; many others contracted illnesses serious enough to require hospitalization. The medical

Conclusion

corps never seemed fully staffed to Spotswood, who characterized his available personnel as being constantly and actively engaged in their duties.

Clearly, much remains unknown about the CSN medical corps, a relatively small and neglected group of men within a comparatively small branch of the Confederate military. Yet the CSN was important to the Southern war effort, and its efficiency was largely influenced by its health. As a group, the officers and enlisted men of the CSN's medical corps served with proficiency and distinction and merit further study.

Appendix A. Commissioned Medical Officers in the CSN

Officer by Initial CSN Grade[a]	CSN Entry Date[b]	Highest Previous Grade[c]	Subsequent Grade(s) CSN	CSA
Surg., Reg. Navy				
Blacknall, George[d,e]	June 14, 1861	Surg., USN	n/p	n/a
Carrington, William F.	Mar. 26, 1861	PAS, USN	n/p	n/a
Conrad, Daniel Burr	June 6, 1861	PAS, USN	n/p	n/a
Cornick, James[d]	Sept. 13, 1861	Surg., USN	n/p	n/a
Fahs, Charles F.[d]	Jan. 1, 1862	Surg., USN	n/p	n/a
Galt, Francis L.	Apr. 15, 1861	PAS, USN	n/p	n/a
Green, Daniel Smith[d,f]	June 22, 1861	Surg., USN	n/p	n/a
Greenhow, James W.B.	Aug. 2, 1861	PAS, USN	n/p	n/a
Harrison, James Francis[d]	June 18, 1861	Surg., USN	n/p	n/a
Harrison, William D.	Mar. 6, 1863	Surg., USN	n/p	n/a
Jeffery, Richard W.[d]	Feb. 8, 1862	Surg., USN	n/p	n/a
Lynah, Arthur Middleton	Mar. 24, 1861	PAS, USN	n/p	n/a
Mason, John T.[d]	June 10, 1861	Surg., USN	n/p	n/a
Mason, Randolph F.[d,g]	June 10, 1861	Surg., USN	n/p	n/a
McClenahan, William F.[d]	June 10, 1861	Surg., USN	n/p	n/a
Minor, Lewis Willis[d]	June 10, 1861	Surg., USN	n/p	n/a
Page, William Meade	Aug. 28, 1862	PAS, USN	n/p	n/a
Patton, William Fairlie[d]	June 10, 1861	Surg. USN	n/p	n/a

Appendix A. Commissioned Medical Officers in the CSN

Officer by Initial CSN Grade[a]	CSN Entry Date[b]	Highest Previous Grade[c]	Subsequent Grade(s) CSN	Subsequent Grade(s) CSA
Phillips, Dinwiddie Brazier[d]	June 10, 1861	PAS, USN	n/p	n/a
Sinclair, William Beverly[d]	June 10, 1861	Surg., USN	n/p	n/a
Spotswood, William A.W.[d]	Mar. 26, 1861	Surg., USN	n/p	n/a
Ward, John[d]	Apr. 20, 1861	PAS, USN	n/p	Surg.[h]
Washington, Henry W.M.	June 18, 1861	PAS, USN	n/p	n/a
Williamson, Charles H.	June 10, 1861	PAS, USN	n/p	n/a
Wysham, William E.[d]	June 10, 1861	PAS, USN	n/p	n/a
Asst. Surg., Reg. Navy				
Charlton, Thomas Jackson, Jr.	Apr. 2, 1861	Asst. Surg., USN	PAS	n/a
Christian, Marcellus P.	July 18, 1861	Asst. Surg., USN	PAS	n/a
Ford, Theodosius Bartow	May 15, 1861	Private, CSA	n/p	n/a
Freeman, Robert J.	Aug. 20, 1861	Asst. Surg., USN	PAS	n/a
Garnett, Algernon S.	June 24, 1861	Asst. Surg., USN	Surg.	n/a
Garretson (Van Bibber), Frederic	June 10, 1861	Asst. Surg., USN	PAS	n/a
Gibbes, Robert Reeve	June 6, 1861	n/a	PAS[i]	n/a
Grafton, Joseph Dana, Jr.[d,j]	June 9, 1861	Asst. Surg., USN	PAS	n/a
Green, Bennett Wood	May 23, 1861	Asst. Surg., USN	PAS	n/a
Griggs, William W.	May 1, 1863	HS, CSA	n/p	n/a
Herty, James W.	Feb. 10, 1862	Asst. Surg., USN	PAS	n/a
Iglehart, Osborn Spriggs	Mar. 27, 1862	Asst. Surg., USN	PAS	n/a
Lindsay, James E.	Jan. 23, 1862	Asst. Surg., USN	PAS	n/a
Lining, Charles E.	Mar. 26, 1861	Asst. Surg., USN	PAS	n/a
Melvin, Henry B.	May 1, 1863	Asst. Surg., CSA	n/p	n/a
Morfit, Charles McLean	June 10, 1861	n/a	PAS[i]	n/a
Parker, Cincinnatus Marion	May 1, 1863	Private, CSA	n/p	n/a
Sandford, John W., Jr.	June 26, 1861	Asst. Surg., USN	PAS	n/a
Stoakley, William S.	May 1, 1863	Asst. Surg., CSA	n/p	n/a
Thomas, Charles Wesley	May 1, 1863	n/a	n/p	n/a
Tipton, Joseph S.	May 1, 1863	Pvt., CSA	n/p	n/a

Appendix A. Commissioned Medical Officers in the CSN

Officer by Initial CSN Grade[a]	CSN Entry Date[b]	Highest Previous Grade[c]	Subsequent Grade(s) CSN	Subsequent Grade(s) CSA
Asst. Surg. for the War, Reg. Navy				
Addison, William J.	April 1, 1862	n/a	Asst. Surg.	n/a
Baldwin, Robert Thomas, Jr.[d]	Mar. 13, 1862	n/a	Asst. Surg.	Asst. Surg.[k]
Belvin, James W.	Feb. 11, 1864	Private, CSA	n/p	n/a
Bondurant, Walter E.	May 10, 1864	Private, CSA	n/p	Asst. Surg.[l]
Bonner, Samuel Lafayette[d]	Mar. 15, 1862	n/a	n/p	Asst. Surg.[m]
Booth, Edwin G.	Apr. 1, 1862	HS, CSA	Asst. Surg.	n/a
Bowles, Richard Curd	Feb. 26, 1863	HS, CSA	Asst. Surg.	n/a
Boxley, James Garland	May 10, 1864	AAS, CSA	n/p	n/a
Brown, Pike	Aug. 31, 1863	Asst. Surg., CSA	n/p	n/a
Caire, Edward	Jan. 7, 1864	n/a	n/p	n/a
Christmas, Henry[d,n]	Mar. 26, 1863	Asst. Surg., CSA	Asst. Surg.	n/a
Claiborne, Gregory Weldon	July 15, 1863	Asst. Surg., CSA	n/p	n/a
Cook, James Valentine	Aug. 30, 1863	Asst. Surg, CSA	Asst. Surg.	n/a
DeBree, John, Jr.	July 18, 1862	n/a	Asst. Surg.	n/a
Dickinson, Luther R.	Jan. 7, 1864	HS, CSA	n/p	n/a
Drewry, Samuel Davies[d,o]	Mar. 26, 1862	n/a	n/p	n/a
Duffel, John E.	May 10, 1864	Asst. Surg., CSA	n/p	n/a
Edmunds, Nicholas C.	Aug. 5, 1862	n/a	Asst. Surg.	n/a
Emory, Thomas	Mar. 15, 1862	n/a	Asst. Surg.	n/a
Ewart, David E.[p]	Jan. 7, 1864	Surg., CSA	n/p	n/a
Foote, George A.	Jan 7, 1864	Asst. Surg., CSA	n/p	n/a

Appendix A. Commissioned Medical Officers in the CSN

Officer by Initial CSN Grade[a]	CSN Entry Date[b]	Highest Previous Grade[c]	Subsequent Grade(s) CSN	Subsequent Grade(s) CSA
Ford, Marcellus	Mar. 11, 1862	n/a	Asst. Surg.	n/a
Goldsborough, Edmund K.	May 10, 1864	n/a	n/p	n/a
Grant, James O.	Aug. 31, 1863	AAS, CSA	Asst. Surg.	n/a
Graves, William W.	Apr. 7, 1862	n/a	Asst. Surg.	n/a
Halstead, George N.	July 15, 1863	HS, CSA	Asst. Surg.	n/a
Harris, Jeptha V.	Jan. 7, 1864	Asst. Surg., CSA	n/p	n/a
Harrison, John C.	Feb. 26, 1863	AAS, CSA	Asst. Surg.	Asst. Surg.[l]
Henderson, Nathaniel K.	Feb. 11, 1864	n/a	n/p	n/a
Herrick, Stephen Solon	Nov. 21, 1862	Asst. Surg, CSA	Asst. Surg.	n/a
Hicks, James M.	Aug. 31, 1863	Private, CSA	n/p	n/a
Jones, William C.	Mar. 26, 1863	n/a	Asst. Surg.	n/a
King, Joel George	Jan. 7, 1864	n/a	n/p	n/a
Kuykendall, Robert C.	Feb. 11, 1864	HS, CSA	n/p	n/a
Land, Henry G.	Aug. 31, 1863	Asst. Surg., CSA	n/p	n/a
Leyburn, John	Jan. 8, 1863	AAS, CSA	Asst. Surg.	n/a
Lipscomb, John Pleasant	Mar. 26, 1863	Private, CSA	Asst. Surg.	n/a
Meade, Hodijah Baylies[d,n]	Feb. 26, 1863	Asst. Surg., CSA	n/p	n/a
Moyler, James Edward	May 10, 1864	Private, CSA	n/p	n/a
Paisley, Hugh S.	May 10, 1864	Asst. Surg., CSA	n/p	n/a
Peck, Frederick	May 10, 1864	AAS, CSA	n/p	n/a
Powell, Robert C.	Jan. 8, 1863	HS, CSA	Asst. Surg.	n/a
Read, Nathaniel Manson	Nov. 26, 1862	Asst. Surg., CSA	Asst. Surg.	n/a

Appendix A. Commissioned Medical Officers in the CSN

Officer by Initial CSN Grade[a]	CSN Entry Date[b]	Highest Previous Grade[c]	Subsequent Grade(s) CSN	Subsequent Grade(s) CSA
Rutherford, John B.	Jan. 7, 1864	Private, CSA	n/p	n/a
Sheppardson, William	Mar. 26, 1863	Asst. Surg, CSA	Asst. Surg.	n/a
Steinriede, John Joseph[q]	Aug. 22, 1862	SS, CSN	n/p	n/a
Stone, Henry[d]	Feb. 26, 1863	AAS, CSA	Asst. Surg.	AAS[r]
Thomas, James Grey	May 10, 1864	Surg., CSA	n/p	n/a
Turner, William Mason	Mar. 13, 1862	Asst. Surg., CSA	Asst. Surg.	n/a
Warner, Watkins L.	Feb. 11, 1864	n/a	n/p	n/a
Weston, George B.	Aug. 31, 1863	n/a	Asst. Surg.	n/a
Williams, William T.[d,s]	Feb. 11, 1864	Colonel, CSA	n/p	n/a
Asst. Surg., PNCS				
Coggin, William W.	Nov. 23, 1864	Asst. Surg., CSA	n/p	n/a
Daniel, George Crawford	Sept. 6, 1864	Private, CSA	n/p	n/a
Sale, William D.	Nov. 23, 1864	HS, CSA	n/p	n/a
Smith, Ira E.	Nov. 23, 1864	Asst. Surg., CSA	n/p	n/a
Sussdorff, Gustave E.	Nov. 23, 1864	n/a	n/p	n/a
Tucker, John H.	Nov. 28, 1864	AAS, CSA	n/p	n/a
Venable, Howell A.	Sept. 6, 1864	AAS, CSA	n/p	n/a
Wheeden, Thomas J.	Oct. 18, 1864	n/a	n/p	n/a

Note: CSN = Confederate States Navy, CSA = Confederate States Army, USN = United States Navy, n/p = not promoted in CSN, n/a = not applicable (did not serve in USN, US Army, CSA, or CSN before appointment as a CSN medical officer. or in the CSA after such appointment), PAS = passed assistant surgeon, HS = hospital steward, AAS = acting assistant surgeon (contract surgeon), SS = surgeon's steward, PNCS = Provisional Navy of the Confederate States. Sources: CSND, *Confederate States Navy Register for 1862*; CSND, *Register of the Officers* (1862); CSND, *Register ... to January 1, 1863*; CSDN, *Register ... to January 1, 1864*; Nominations and confirmations, JCCSA; Compiled service records, microfilm M331, RG 109. Information was also obtained from newspapers, published biographies, and other sources.

[a]Names, as they usually appear in CSN documents, have been expanded or corrected. Unless otherwise noted, (1) officers in the regular CSN were appointed to the PNCS at a grade identical to their final grade in the regular CSN, and (2) promotions were restricted to the regular CSN.

Appendix A. Commissioned Medical Officers in the CSN

[b]Date pertains to service as an officer and is the earliest of an individual's acceptance of his appointment, original entry into service, congressional approval of his appointment, or the "to rank from" (seniority) date given in his appointment.

[c]Previous military duty may have been separated from CSN appointment by a period of civilian life. Service in state navies is not included.

[d]Not appointed to the PNCS.

[e]Died January 21, 1862.

[f]Died March 5, 1864.

[g]Died August 9, 1862.

[h]Resigned from the CSN December 5, 1862, before entering the CSA.

[i]Promoted to PAS in the PNCS in November 1864 without congressional record of also being promoted in the regular CSN.

[j]Died May 29, 1863.

[k]Resigned from the CSN July 25, 1863, before entering the CSA.

[l]No documentation of resignation from CSN has been found.

[m]Resigned from the CSN August 20, 1862, before entering the CSA.

[n]Declined CSN appointment(s).

[o]Resigned from the CSN in fall 1862.

[p]Died October 11, 1864.

[q]Steinriede was appointed by the president on August 22, 1862, as an "acting assistant surgeon for the war," but "assistant surgeon for the war" was probably meant. He resigned from the CSN on February 17, 1863.

[r]Resigned from the CSN on August 26, 1863, before entering CSA.

[s]Died March 9, 1864.

Appendix B.
Duties of Medical Officers

(from CSND, *Regulations*, 122–29)

CHAPTER XVII.
FLEET SURGEON.

ARTICLE 1. *Duties of a fleet surgeon.* The fleet surgeon is to have a general supervision over all medical officers of the squadron to which he may be attached, and he will report to the commander-in-chief any neglect of duty that may come under his notice. He is charged with receiving and forwarding (through the prescribed channels) all communications and reports from medical officers for the Bureau of Medicine and Surgery, and with the examination and approval of all requisitions and bills for the medical department, and procuring supplies from the depots or naval storekeepers abroad, and with purchasing them when the required supplies cannot be otherwise obtained.

ARTICLE 2. *To co-operate with the Chief of the Bureau of Medicine and Surgery.* The fleet surgeon is expected to co-operate with the Chief of the Bureau of Medicine and Surgery, by close attention to the duties of his own office and to those placed under his supervision, and to secure proper economy and promptness and punctuality in making and forwarding reports and returns.

ARTICLE 3. *Prevention of disease.* He will suggest to the commander-in-chief, for his consideration, proper measures for preventing or checking disease, or for promoting the comfort of the sick or wounded.

ARTICLE 4. *He will specify vessels whose crews are least fit for active service.* He will, when required by the commander-in-chief, specify those vessels which may appear, from the state of the health of the crews, least fit for active service, or requiring change of climate or diet.

ARTICLE 5. *Persons unfit for the cruise, and deteriorated articles to be reported.* He will report to the commanding officer such officers and persons of inferior ratings as he may deem unfit for the cruise, with a view to a survey on them; and when out of the Confederate States, such articles as in his opinion have deteriorated, and with the approval of the commanding officer he will detail the medical officers for surveys.

Appendix B. Duties of Medical Officers

ARTICLE 6. *Journal of daily practice.* He will keep a journal of daily practice, according to such form as may be prescribed by the Bureau of Medicine and Surgery; inspect the like journals of the other surgeons of the fleet, and make such suggestions to the surgeon in charge as he may deem proper.

ARTICLE 7. *Note-book.* He will keep a *note-book* in addition to his journal, in such form as the Chief of the Bureau of Medicine and Surgery may prescribe, in which he will record such matters of interest as my come under his notice in relation to climate, disease, medical statistics, and any other professional matter.

ARTICLE 8. *Disposition of journal and note-book.* His journal and note-book, with those of the other surgeons, will be transmitted to the department at such periods as the Secretary of the Navy may direct through the prescribed channels.

CHAPTER XVIII.
SURGEON.

ARTICLE 1. *He will take charge of all medicines, &c.* A surgeon will, on joining a vessel, navy yard, or hospital, for duty, take charge of and receipt for all medicines, surgical instruments, and hospital stores.

ARTICLE 2. *He will conform to regulations and allowances of medicines.* He will conform to the regulations, and to such allowances of medicines, instruments, and stores as may be established by the Bureau of Medicine and Surgery, when making requisitions, unless there should be some special cause for varying from them, when such cause must be stated upon the requisition.

ARTICLE 3. *Account of receipts and expenditures.* He will keep a regular account of receipts and expenditures in his department, according to such forms as may be prescribed by the Bureau of Medicine and Surgery, and when on sea duty will make quarterly reports of hospital stores expended and on hand to his commanding officer.

ARTICLE 4. *He will be allowed a store-room.* He will be allowed, to his exclusive use, a convenient store-room for the preservation of articles in his charge.

ARTICLE 5. *He will be attentive to cleanliness and supply of medicines.* He will be attentive to the cleanliness of the sick, their bedding and the sick bay, and will take special care that the sick are supplied at proper times with the medicine and food their condition may require.

ARTICLE 6. *Daily report to the commanding officer.* He will report to the commanding officer, daily, the names and condition of the sick, according to such forms as may be prescribed; and will, at the same time, suggest any measures he may deem important for the health of the crew.

ARTICLE 7. *Binnacle list.* He will cause to be deposited daily, in the binnacle, a list of the officers and other persons whose condition requires that they should be excused from duty, or whose allowance of spirits is temporarily stopped.

Appendix B. Duties of Medical Officers

ARTICLE 8. *Infections disease.* He will take all possible precautions to prevent the introduction or progress of any infectious disease, and make immediate report to the commander of any probable danger from, or the appearance of, any such disease.

ARTICLE 9. *Examination of the men when they join the vessel.* He is carefully to examine the crew as soon as practicable after joining the ship, for the purpose of reporting to the commanding officer any necessity that may exist for vaccination, which, if possible, is to be performed before the sailing of the vessel.

ARTICLE 10. *Persons to assist in preparing food for the sick.* He will, upon application to the commanding officer, be allowed proper persons to assist in the preparation of articles for the nourishment of the sick, and to perform other services for their comfort.

ARTICLE 11. *To be prepared to relieve wounded.* He is at all times to have in readiness everything necessary for the relief of the wounded.

ARTICLE 12. *Tourniquets to be distributed prior to an engagement.* On the probability of an engagement, he will cause a sufficient number of tourniquets to be distributed to the officers, in different parts of the ship, and see that all persons stationed with him, and such others as may be designated, are instructed in the proper mode of using them.

ARTICLE 13. *Sick sent to hospital.* When practicable, sick persons who may be sent to a hospital, or hospital vessel, are to be accompanied by a medical officer, and the surgeon will send with them a statement of their diseases or injuries, with a synopsis of treatment, according to such forms as may be prescribed by the Bureau of Medicine and Surgery.

ARTICLE 14. *Examination of articles in bumboats.* He will cause the boats attending the ship with article of food for sale, to be examined, and if any contain articles the use of which would, in his opinion, in injurious to the crew, he will represent the same to the commanding officer.

ARTICLE 15. *Journal of daily practice.* He will keep a journal of daily practice according to such form as may be prescribed by the Bureau of Medicine and Surgery. The journal to be subject, if required, to the inspection of the surgeon of the fleet, and to be forwarded, as directed for correspondence and other reports, for deposit with the chief of the Bureau of Medicine and Surgery, through the proper channels.

ARTICLE 16. *Note Book.* He shall, in addition to a journal of daily practice, keep a note book similar to that prescribed in article 7 of chapter XVII., and forward it as provided for in article 8 of the same chapter.

ARTICLE 17. *Return of the articles in his charge when the ship is placed in ordinary.* When the ship is placed in ordinary he will return into the proper store all articles remaining in his charge, and will be held strictly accountable for any deficiency or injury that may not be satisfactorily accounted for.

ARTICLE 18. *Reports and surveys on persons who receive wounds that*

Appendix B. Duties of Medical Officers

may entitle them to pensions. Whenever any person on board shall receive any wound or injury which may probably entitle him to make application for a pension, the surgeon shall report the same to the commander, in writing, before the person be removed or discharged from the vessel, that a proper survey may be held, and certificate issued, according to such form as may be prescribed by the Pension Office.

ARTICLE 19. *Persons left in hospital.* When petty officers or persons of inferior rating are left in a hospital after the sailing of a vessel from when they were sent, the surgeon of the hospital must report to the commander of the station whenever any of them are in a situation to justify their removal, that they may be sent to some other vessel or discharged.

ARTICLE 20. *Reports on persons in hospital who are convalescent.* If any petty officer or person of inferior rating shall not have so far recovered as to justify his removal from the hospital when his time of service shall have expired, or in the injuries or disease of any person sent to the hospital will, in the opinion of the surgeon, prove incurable or produce long-continued inability to perform duty, the surgeon must immediately report such cases to the commander of the station, making a particular statement of all the facts and circumstances connected with each case within his knowledge, that they may be transmitted to the Secretary of the Navy for his decision.

CHAPTER XIX.
PASSED AND OTHER ASSISTANT SURGEONS.

ARTICLE 1. *They shall see that medicines are properly prepared.* Assistant surgeons, whether passed or otherwise, and when no assistant surgeon, the surgeon shall attend personally to see that medicines are properly prepared and labelled for distribution to the sick. [*Author's note*: The intended meaning is "...whether passed or otherwise—and when there is no passed or other assistant surgeon, then the surgeon—shall attend...," as inferred from Code of Regulations, in *Report of the Secretary of the Navy*, Dec. 6, 1858, H.R. Exec. Doc. 2, 35th Cong., 2nd sess., 130 (1858)].

ARTICLE 2. *They shall perform the duties assigned to them, and conform to orders.* They shall perform all the professional duties which may be given by the surgeon of the vessel, navy yard, or hospital, to which they may be attached; and will be unremitting in their attentions to the comfort and cleanliness of the sick, and exact from those under their direction a rigid performance of their duties.

ARTICLE 3. *The oldest passed or other assistant surgeon will perform the duties of surgeon.* In the absence of the surgeon, the passed or other assistant surgeon oldest in commission, is to perform all the duties of the surgeon.

Chapter Notes

Works, designators, and institutional authors frequently cited in the notes are identified by the following abbreviations and short forms:

CSND: Confederate States Navy Department
Gibbes diary: Diary of Dr. Robert Reeve Gibbes, 1861–1865, National Civil War Naval Museum
JCCSA: *Journal of the Congress of the Confederate States of America, 1861–1865*
MR: Miscellaneous Records of the Office of Naval Records and Library, microfilm T829, RG 45
OR: *War of the Rebellion: A Compilation of the Official Records of the Union and Confederate Armies*
ORN: *Official Records of the Union and Confederate Navies in the War of the Rebellion*
RG: Record Group, National Archives and Records Administration
SF: Subject File of the Confederate States Navy, microfilm M1091, RG 45
USND: United States Navy Department

Foreword

1. Silverstone, *Civil War Navies*, ix, 4–12, 111–18; Canney, *Lincoln's Navy*, 17; Porter, *Naval History of the Civil War*, 18, 36, 37, 465, 680–81.
2. Campbell, *Confederate Ironclads at War*, 1–3, 44–57; Silverstone, *Civil War Navies*, 149–92; Still, *Confederate Navy*, 31–33, 38–39; Canney, *Lincoln's Navy*, 18–19; Luraghi, *History of the Confederate Navy*, 33; Scharf, *History of the Confederate States Navy*, 47; Dufour, *Night the War Was Lost*, 335–38.
3. Blum and DeBruyne, American War and Military Operations Casualties, 2; Sullivan, *Marines of the Civil War*, 186–202; Lynch, "Confederate Navy Medicine," 811; Lynch, "Civil War Federal Navy Physicians," 1046.
4. Lynch, "Confederate Navy Medicine," 811–12; Lynch, "Civil War Federal Navy Physicians," 1046; Blum and DeBruyne, American War and Military Operations Casualties, 2; Farragut to Gideon Welles, July 20, 1862, *ORN*, ser. 1, 19:80–81; Davis to Welles, July 23, 1862, *ORN*, ser. 1, 19:48–49; Kenney, "From the Log of the Red Rover."
5. Hasegawa, *Matchless Organization*.

Preface

1. Chitwood, "Doctor Spotswood"; Lynch, "Confederate Navy Medicine"; Tomblin, *Life in Jefferson Davis' Navy*.

Introduction

1. Luraghi, *History of the Confederate Navy*, 2–7.
2. Resolution, Feb. 14, 1861, *JCCSA*, 1:51; Report of Committee on Naval Affairs, Feb. 1861, *ORN*, ser. 2, 2:41.
3. Act of Feb. 21, 1861, ch. 10, Prov. Cong. C.S.A. Stat. 33 (1864); Mallory resignation, Jan. 21, 1861, *Cong. Globe*, 36th

Notes—Chapter 1

Cong., 2nd sess., 485–86 (1861); Mallory committee appointment, Dec. 8. 1851, S. Journal, 32nd Cong., 1st sess., 34–35 (1852); Mallory committee chairmanship, Dec. 13, 1855, S. Journal, 34th Cong., 1st sess., 14 (1856); Mallory confirmation, Mar. 4, 1861, *JCCSA*, 1:106. The unicameral Provisional Congress existed from February 4, 1861, to February 17, 1862. The bicameral Confederate Congress began its first session on February 18, 1862.

4. John K. Mitchell to Mallory, Apr., 28, 1864, *ORN*, ser. 2, 2:753–55; 739–41; Mallory to Jefferson Davis, Apr. 30, 1864, *ORN*, ser. 2 2:630–39.

5. Davis to Congress, *OR*, ser. 4, 1: 950–52.

Chapter 1

1. Act of Feb. 9, 1861, ch. 1, Prov. Cong. C.S.A. Stat. 27 (1864); Act of Mar. 16, 1861, ch. 58, Prov. Cong. C.S.A. Stat. 70 (1864); Act of Aug. 31, 1842, ch. 286, 5 Stat. 579 (1856); Scharf, *History of the Confederate States Navy*, 29–30. The USN divisions were called bureaus. The analogous CSN divisions were called bureaus in CSN regulations but were most commonly called offices. Mallory referred to the various offices four days before the act creating them was approved. At that time, he did not call the offices by their eventual names (Mallory, cost estimates, Mar. 12, 1861, entry 160, RG 109).

2. Act of Aug. 31, 1842, ch. 286, 5 Stat. 579 (1856); Act of Mar. 16, 1861, ch. 58, Prov. Cong. C.S.A. Stat. 70 (1864). During the Civil War, *grade* most properly referred to a tier in the military hierarchy and was denoted by a title such as captain, commander, surgeon, or assistant surgeon. *Rank* was the relative and unique place that an officer held among other officers. Within a particular grade, the officer with the most seniority—determined by the date of his commissions—held the highest rank. All officers within a particular grade outranked all officers of lower grades. In the seniority system, the officer with the highest rank would be the first to be promoted to the next grade when a vacancy occurred at the higher grade.

3. USND, *Instructions for the Government* (1857), 3; Abel P. Upshur, *Report of the Secretary of the Navy*, Dec. 1842, H.R. Exec. Doc. 2, 27th Cong., 3rd sess., 538 (1842). The first edition of *Instructions for the Government* was published in 1844.

4. Homans, *Register*, 10; Langley, *History of Medicine in the Early U.S. Navy*, 357; USND, *Register* (1845), 22; Whelan confirmation, Jan. 23, 1854, *S. Exec. Journal*, 33rd Cong., 1st sess., 168–69, 215 (1887).

5. USND, *Register* (1853), 16, 46–50; Frederick Horner, "Medical Corps of the U.S. Navy."

6. Mallory, cost estimates, Mar. 12, 1861, entry 160, RG 109; CSND, *Register... to January 1, 1864*, 12–13; CSND, *Instructions for the Guidance*, 3.

7. Chitwood, "Doctor Spotswood"; "First Alumnus"; Naval Register for the Year 1830, January 4, 1830, *American State Papers: Naval Affairs* 3:402–36; USND, *Register* (1861), 38; Abstract 965, roll 9, microfilm M330, RG 24; Spotswood to Isaac Toucey, Jan. 19, 1861, roll 390, MR; Spotswood to Andrew Johnson, June 28, 1865, roll 15, microfilm M1003, RG 94; CSND, *Register... to January 1, 1863*; Payroll, Pensacola Navy Yard, Apr. 1861, roll 165, MR. The Pensacola Navy Yard and Naval Hospital were closer to Warrington, Florida, than to Pensacola and were sometimes referred to as the Warrington Navy Yard and Naval Hospital.

8. Chitwood, "Doctor Spotswood"; Thomas Chalmers McCorvey, "An Unheralded Battle—One of the Last Conflicts of the War between the States," *Montgomery (AL) Advertiser*, Sept. 10, 1911, 23; Spotswood to Bledsoe, Sept. 12, 1861, roll 41, microfilm M251, RG 109; CSND, *Register... to January 1, 1863*; File for Thomas E. Spotwood [sic], roll 452, microfilm M311, RG 109.

9. Mary G. Spotswood to Christopher G. Memminger, Feb. 9, 1864, and to

Notes—Chapter 1

unknown, roll 972, microfilm M346, RG 109; Mary G. Spotswood to Cooper, Oct. 11, 1864, with endorsement, roll 145, microfilm M474, RG 109; Provision Fund Receipt, n.d., file for Lizzie Archer, roll 21, microfilm M346, RG 109.

10. Spotswood to Bledsoe, Sept. 12, 1861, roll 41, microfilm M251, RG 109; Invoice for E.B. Wheelock, May 3, 1861, and for Thiess and Pollard, May 23, 1861, roll 14, SF; Mallory, cost estimates, Mar. 12, 1861, entry 160, RG 109; Mallory, cost estimate, Apr. 28, 1861, *ORN*, ser. 2, 2:57. Although Carrington was in Montgomery in May 1861, he was paid at Pensacola for services during May and June 1861 (Payrolls, Warrington Navy Yard, roll 165, MR). A receiving ship was a vessel docked at a harbor and used to recruit sailors and prepare them for naval service.

11. Jones, *Rebel War Clerk's Diary*, vol. 1, 32; Vanfelson, *Little Red Book*, 10–11; *Stranger's Guide*, 14; De Leon, *Belles Beaux and Brains*, 251; Charles E.L. Stuart [Col. C.S. Armee, pseud.], "Rummaging through Rebeldom: Sixteenth Rummage" and "Rummaging through Rebeldom: Nineteenth Rummage," *New York Citizen*, July 20, 1867, 1–2, and Aug. 10, 1867, 2. C.E.L. Stuart, a former Confederate Navy Department clerk, described the department offices as being on the first floor of the Virginia Mechanics Institute building, but in his nomenclature, the first floor was the level above the ground floor.

12. Mallory to Jefferson Davis, Feb. 12, 1862, in Davis, Message to the President of the Congress; CSND, *Register ... to January 1, 1863*; CSND, *Register... to January 1, 1864*; 1860 U.S. Census, Escambia County, FL, population schedule, city of Pensacola, p. 373 (21 penned), dwelling 160, family 160, Charles and Robert Fennell, roll 106, microfilm M653, RG 29; James S. Jones to James M. Baker, Mar. 25, 1865, file for Jones, roll 522, microfilm M346, RG 109; Voucher for Robert A. Fennell, Nov. 30, 1863, microfilm roll 14, SF; Spotswood to Mallory, Nov. 1, 1864, *ORN*, ser. 2, 2:758–60; Hasegawa, *Matchless Organization*, 190–92.

13. Spotswood to Bledsoe, Sept. 12, 1861, roll 41, microfilm M251, RG 109; Voucher for Purcell, Ladd & Co., Nov. 29, 1861, roll 15, SF; Voucher for I.C. Du Bose & Co., Oct. 24, 1862, and for Tom Griffin, Feb. 2, 1863, roll 14, SF. French Forrest to Jeffery, Nov. 8, 1862, ZB file for Jeffery, Navy Department Library.

14. Petition of Dental Surgeons (Senate petition D.4), Dec. 29, 1863, entry 175, RG 109; Voucher for C. Polvogt, Dec. 15, 1863, for W.H. Lippitt, Dec. 31, 1864, and for Wilson Temple, Jan. 1, 1864, roll 15, SF; Voucher for Thomas R. Ware, Sept. 30, 1864, roll 14, SF.

15. Jeffery, cost estimate, Dec. 16, 1862, and Harrison, cost estimate, Feb. 22, 1865, entry 160, RG 109; Spotswood to Andrew Johnson, June 28, 1865, roll 15, microfilm M1003, RG 94.

16. Code of Regulations, in *Report of the Secretary of the Navy*, Dec. 6, 1858, H.R. Exec. Doc. 2, 35th Cong., 2nd sess., 24–430 (1858); CSND, *Regulations*; USND, *Instructions for the Government* (1857); CSND, *Instructions for the Guidance*. The Confederate *Instructions*, dated November 1, 1862, were published in Richmond in 1864, but they were evidently available in printed form by December 1862, when 100 copies were purchased for the CSN hospital in Richmond (invoice for Purcell, Ladd & Co., Dec. 12, 1862, roll 15, SF). Although the U.S. Attorney General had ruled in 1853 that various prewar issuances of the USN were invalid as regulations, a code of regulations, cited above, was introduced in 1858 and is assumed to have been the basis of CSN regulations. In 1862, the U.S. Congress recognized the 1858 code of regulations, and other issuances, as constituting the USN regulations (C. Cushing to James C. Dobbins, Apr. 5, 1853, in *Report of the Secretary of the Navy*, H.R. Exec. Doc. 2, 35th Cong., 2nd sess., 24–430 [1858]; Act of July 14, 1862, ch. 164, § 5, 12 Stat. 561, 565 [1863]).

17. Hasegawa, *Matchless Organization*, 155–57; Freeman, *Calendar of Confederate Papers*, 33–34; "Association of Army and Navy Surgeons."

18. Hasegawa, *Matchless Organi-*

Notes—Chapter 2

zation, 157–59; Jeffery, "Gun-shot Wound of Lung, Liver and Intestines."

19. Spotswood to Mallory, Nov. 30, 1863, Apr. 28, 1864, and Nov. 1, 1864, *ORN*, ser. 2, 2:559–63, 647, 758–62.

Chapter 2

1. Act of Mar. 16, 1861, ch. 58, Prov. Cong. C.S.A. Stat. 70 (1864); Resolution, Feb. 13, 1861, *JCCSA*, 1:48.
2. Act of Mar. 16, 1861, ch. 58, Prov. Cong. C.S.A. Stat. 70 (1864); Wells, *Confederate Navy*, 19–20; Mallory to Davis, Apr. 26, 1861, *ORN*, ser. 2, 2:51–55; CSND, *Register of the Officers* (1862), 7. The CSN register for 1862 shows Charlton accepting his appointment as CSN assistant surgeon on April 20, 1861, which is consistent with his congressional confirmation on May 21, 1861. The CSN registers for 1863 and 1864 show Charlton's original service date as April 2, 1862. Lynah's name was often misspelled as Lynch.
3. Isaac Toucey to Charlton, Dec. 18, 1860, roll 390, MF; Charlton to H.C. Wayne, Feb. 20, 1861, Incoming Correspondence, Adjutant General, document 22-1-17, Georgia State Archives; CSND, *Register ... to January 1, 1863*, 10. Dates denoting the start of Confederate service are, when available, taken from the 1863 and 1864 CSN registers. Such dates often preceded the dates on which the Confederate Congress approved the officers' appointments.
4. USND, *Register* (1855), 48; USND, *Register* (1858), 100; Brown to Leroy P. Walker, May 2, 1861, roll 47, microfilm M331, RG 109; Act of May 20, 1861, ch. 32, Prov. Cong. C.S.A. Stat 121 (1864); Mallory to Jefferson Davis, July 18, 1861, *ORN*, ser. 2, 2:76–79; "Appointments by the Governor by and with the Advice and Consent of the Military Board," *Weekly Standard* (Raleigh, NC), May 22, 1861, 4; Compiled service record for Brown, roll 249, microfilm M270, RG 109.
5. Callahan, *List of Officers*, 212; "The Confederate Congress," *Daily Richmond Examiner*, July 27, 1861, 2; Robertson, *Proceedings of the Advisory Council*, 99;

Garnett to Andrew Johnston, May 7[?], 1867, roll 73, microfilm M1003, RG 94.

6. USND, *Registers* (1856–60); USND, *Register* (1863), 109, 113–14.
7. Dudley, *Going South*; Parker, "Confederate States Navy," 4; Scharf, *History of the Confederate States Navy*, 606.
8. Williamson to James Speed, June 1, 1865, roll 71, microfilm M1003, RG 94.
9. Harrison to Andrew Johnson, July 6, 1865, roll 162, microfilm M1003, RG 94; USND, *Register* (1864), 113; CSND, *Register ... to January 1, 1864*, 12.
10. Statements for Cornick (p. 21) and Greenhow (p. 171), entry 43, RG 52; Act of Feb. 21, 1861, ch. 49, § 3, 12 Stat. 147, 150 (1863); CSND, *Register ... to January 1, 1863*, 10–11; CSND, *Register ... to January 1, 1864*, 12–13, 43.
11. Jeffery to Welles, July 12, 1861, Page to Welles, July 16, 1861, and Lindsay to Welles, July 16, 1861, roll 389, MF; Welles to Jeffery, Sept. 28, 1861, Welles to Page, Oct. 10, 1861, and Welles to Lindsay, Oct. 10, 1861, roll 390, MF; Jeffery to Lorenzo Thomas, Dec. 20, 1861, file J236, roll 32, microfilm M619, RG 94; List of Prisoners of State at Fort Warren, Boston Harbor, Nov. 27, 1861, *OR*, ser. 2, 2:154; William F. Martin to Judah P. Benjamin, Dec. 27, 1861, *OR*, ser. 2, 3:762–63; Benjamin to John H. Winder, Jan. 24, 1862, *OR*, ser. 2, 3:277–78; CSND, *Register ... to January 1, 1863*, 10.
12. Act of May 20, 1861, ch. 32, Prov. Cong. C.S.A. Stat 121 (1864); Mallory to Davis, July 18, 1861, *ORN*, ser. 2, 2:76–79; CSND, *Register ... to January 1, 1863*, 10; USND, *Register* (1861); Nominations, July 30, 1861, *JCCSA*, 1:298. Naval registers typically showed the state in which officers were born, from which they were appointed, and in which they were a citizen; the latter two entries could differ for the same man between USN and CSN registers.
13. Compiled service record for Ford, roll 195, microfilm M266, RG 109; News item, *Daily Chronicle & Sentinel* (Augusta, GA), May 18, 1861, 3; Ford appointment, May 21, 1861, *JCCSA*, 1:266–67.
14. Entries for Gibbes (no. 1713) and Morfit (no. 1792), entry 137, RG 45; Morfit

and Gibbes nominations, July 30, 1861, *JCCSA*, 1:298; "Medical Service, United States Navy"; Gibbes diary, Sept. 4, 1863; Entry for Morfit (no. 1141½), roll 9, microfilm M330, RG 24; Statement for Morfit (p. 22), entry 43, RG 52; Butcher, *Genealogical and Personal History*, 1299–1300; "Deaths"; Robertson, *Proceedings of the Advisory Council*, 98; CSND, *Register ... to January 1, 1863*; An Ordinance Establishing the Navy of Virginia, Apr. 27, 1861, *Ordinances Adopted by the Convention of Virginia*, 8–9.

15. Robertson, *Proceedings of the Advisory Council*, 2, 40–41, 69, 98, 106, 113, 159, 161, 164; CSND, *Register ... to January 1, 1863*; Statement for Beck, entry 43, RG 52, p. 251; Entries for Beck, USND, *Register* (1854–61, 1863); "Dr. Beck," *Daily Dispatch* (Richmond), May 8, 1861, 3. Harrison was nominated as a Passed Assistant Surgeon in the Virginia navy on June 18, 1861, even though he knew of his promotion on March 15, 1861, to surgeon in the USN. He was dismissed from the USN on July 29, 1861, after tendering his resignation on June 15, 1861 (Harrison to Gideon Welles, Mar. 29, 1861, roll 272, microfilm M148, RG 45; Welles to Harrison, July 29, 1861, roll 390, MF).

16. Gibbes diary, Jan. 7–May 27, 1861; "South Carolina Navy," *Charleston Daily Courier*, Apr. 25, 1861, 2; "A Vessel Stopped," *Charleston Daily Courier*, May 21, 1861; Prize money distribution, Dec. 31, 1861, roll 171, MF; Pelot army appointment, *JCCSA*, 3:543; Robertson, *Proceedings of the Advisory Council*, 99; Warren, *Doctor's Experiences*, 266.

17. Day, "Leon Smith"; CSN Prisoners of War, roll 16, SF; J.R. Marmion to E.P. Turner, Sept. 12, 1863, file for Barnett, roll 16, microfilm M331, RG 109; J.N. Barney to S.R. Mallory, Mar. 9, 1863, *ORN*, ser. 1, 19:849–50; George F. Emmons to Gideon Welles, Dec. 29, 1864, *ORN*, ser. 1, 21:777–78.

18. Gideon Welles to H. Hamlin, Dec. 29, 1863, S. Exec. Doc. 3, 38th Cong., 1st sess., 1864, 8–9; CSND, *Register ... to January 1, 1863*; CSND, *Register ... to January 1, 1864*; Dudley, *Going South*;

"Dr. Thomas B. Steele," *Sun* (Baltimore), June 23, 1905, 10; "Dr. Charles Lowndes, of Talbot, is Dead," *Baltimore American*, Feb. 25, 1920, 2.

Chapter 3

1. Act of Dec. 24, 1861, ch. 24, Prov. Cong. C.S.A. Stat. 229 (1864).

2. CSND, *Register ... to January 1, 1863*, 12; Drewry to Andrew Johnson, Oct. 16, 1865, roll 59, microfilm M1003, RG 94; Act of Apr. 16, 1862, ch. 31, Cong. C.S.A. Stat. 29 (1862); Act of Oct. 11, 1862, ch. 45, Cong. C.S.A. Stat. 77 (1862); Muster roll, *Patrick Henry*, roll 179, MF; Muster and pay rolls, Drewry's Bluff, roll 172, MF.

3. Cornick, Announcement, *Daily Dispatch* (Richmond), Feb. 27, 1862, 1; Cornick, Announcement, *Charleston Daily Courier*, Apr. 28, 1862, 2; Cornick, Announcement, *Daily Richmond Examiner*, Apr. 2, 1864, 3; Minor, Announcement, *Richmond Whig and Public Advertiser*, Sept. 18, 1862, 3.

4. Cornick, Announcement, *Charleston Daily Courier* Apr. 28, 1862, 2; Hamilton, *Practical Treatise on Military Surgery*, 222–24.

5. Hamilton, *Practical Treatise on Military Surgery*, 222–24; G.R.B. Horner, *Diseases and Injuries of Seamen*, 26–27, 33–36.

6. Benjamin J. Walker, letter of recommendation, Nov. 9, 1863, file B2630, roll 60, microfilm M474, RG 109; Compiled service records for Bracey, rolls 26 (3rd VA Cav.) and 545 (14th VA Inf.), microfilm M324, RG 109.

7. Gradijan, "Navy Surgeons in the Civil War"; Hasegawa, *Matchless Organization*, 145; Koste, "Medical School for a Nation," 31.

8. Hamilton, *Practical Treatise on Military Surgery*, 222–24; USND, *Regulations*, 36–42; Examination Papers Collection, National Library of Medicine.

9. G.R.B. Horner, *Diseases and Injuries of Seamen*, 26–27, Gradijan, "Navy Surgeons in the Civil War."

10. "Medical Service, United States

Notes—Chapter 3

Navy"; Assistant surgeons, USND, *Register* (1861), 44. Iglehart's name was often misspelled as Inglehart.

11. Hasegawa, "Officers' Promotions"; Mallory to Jefferson Davis, Feb. 27, 1862, *ORN*, ser. 2, 2:149–54; CSND, *Register of the Officers* (1862), 7; CSND, *Register ... to January 1, 1863*, 10; Blacknall death notice, *Richmond Whig and Public Advertiser*, January 24, 1862, 1.

12. Act of April 21, 1862, ch. 68, Cong. C.S.A. Stat 50 (1862); Information from President's Message of Nov. 9, 1864, roll 16, SF; Hamilton, *Practical Treatise on Military Surgery*, 222–24; CSND, *Register ... to January 1, 1864*, 55–56; Appointment of Charlton, Garretson, and Sandford, Sept. 13, 1862, *JCCSA*, 2:281.

13. Hamilton, *Practical Treatise on Military Surgery*, 222–24; CSND, *Register ... to January 1, 1864*, 14–15; Promotions, *JCCSA*, 3:54; 4:144–46.

14. Thomas W. Brent to Sandford, May 26, 1862, and Brent to Charlton, May 29, 1862, ZB files for Sandford and Charlton, Navy Department Library.

15. Gibbes diary, Jan. 12, Jan. 14, Apr. 25, and May 2–9, 1864; John K. Mitchell to Morfit, Apr. 12, 1864, roll 16, SF.

16. Garnett promotion, *JCCSA*, 2:233, 240.

17. CSND, *Register ... to January 1, 1863*; CSND, *Register ... to January 1, 1864*.

18. Spotswood to Mallory, Nov. 30, 1863, *ORN*, ser. 2, 22:559–61.

19. CSND, *Register ... to January 1, 1864*, 14; USND, *Register* (1861), 41–42.

20. Spotswood to Mallory, Apr. 28, 1864, *ORN*, ser. 2, 2:647.

21. Act of May 1, 1863, ch. 85, Cong. C.S.A. Stat. 161 (1863).

22. Nominations and confirmations, *JCCSA*, 4:264, 265, 287, 296.

23. Spotswood to Mallory, Nov. 1, 1864, *ORN*, ser. 2, 2:758–60. In the CSN, a squadron usually consisted of several vessels, under command of a flag officer, assembled for the defense of the coast, seaports, or rivers in a specified geographic area.

24. CSND, *Register... to January 1, 1864*, 12–15; Spotswood to Mallory, Apr. 28, 1864, *ORN*, ser. 2, 2:647.

25. File for Bowles, roll 34, microfilm M347, RG 109; Compiled service records for Bondurant, roll 27, microfilm M331, RG 109, and roll 271, microfilm M324, RG 109; Compiled service records for Harrison, microfilm roll 120, microfilm M331, RG 109, and roll 587, microfilm M324, RG 109. Documentation of army medical service of CSN medical officers can usually be found in their army compiled service records (microfilm M331, RG 109).

26. Thomas to Samuel Cooper, Oct. 27, 1863, with accompanying certificate, roll 245, microfilm M331, RG 109; Paisley to Cooper, May 20, 1863, roll 192, microfilm M331, RG 109; CSND, *Register ... to January 1, 1864*, 44; Voucher for E. & T. Sill, Sept. 9, 1864; roll 15, SF.

27. Hasegawa, *Matchless Organization*, 139–47; File for Coggin, no. C2378, roll 62, microfilm M474, RG 109; Surgeon General's Office, Special Orders, Sept. 24, 1864, file for Coggin, roll 58, microfilm M331, RG 109; Coggin CSN nomination (Nov. 10, 1864) and confirmation (Nov. 23, 1864), *JCCSA*, 4:265, 287. Coggins's middle initial appears as *M*—almost certainly incorrectly—rather than *W*, in the Confederate congressional record of his CSN nomination and appointment.

28. Entries for Dickinson (page 47) and Sale (page 37), vol. 557, ch. 6, RG 109; Hasegawa, *Matchless Organization*, 149–50; Medical College of Virginia statement of graduates, 1863 and 1864, Sanger Historical Files, Tompkins-McCaw Library; Compiled service record for Parker, roll 272, microfilm M269, RG 109.

29. Turner to Judah P. Benjamin, Mar. 2, 1862, file T157, roll 252, microfilm M331, RG 109.

30. CSND, *Register of the Officers* (1862); CSND, *Register ... to January 1, 1863*; CSND, *Register ... to January 1, 1864*; CSN Prisoners of War, roll 16, SF.

31. USND, *Register* (1865); "Volunteer Navy in the Civil War"; Hasegawa, *Matchless Organization*, 18.

Notes—Chapter 4

Chapter 4

1. Ruschenberger, *Brief History*; Paullin, "Naval Administration" 1465–68; Act of Mar. 16, 1861, ch. 58, Prov. Cong. C.S.A. Stat. 70 (1864); Act of Apr. 21, 1862; ch. 68, Cong. C.S.A. Stat. 50 (1862).

2. CSND, *Regulations*, 8; Act of Apr. 21, 1862; ch. 68, Cong. C.S.A. Stat. 50 (1862); Mallory, General Order, Nov. 22, 1862, in CSND, *Register ... to January 1, 1863*, 1; Mitchell to James W. Robertson, Apr. 1, 1864, roll 14, microfilm M625, RG 45.

3. USND, *Uniform and Dress of the Navy of the Confederate States*; Gibbes diary, Apr. 4, 1863.

4. Act of Mar. 16, 1861, ch. 58, Prov. Cong. C.S.A. Stat. 70 (1864); Ruschenberger, *Brief History*, 15; Medical Officers of the Confederate States, Broadside, n.d., call no. 186-: 5, Broadside Collection, Virginia Museum of History and Culture; Act of Feb. 16, 1864, ch. 40, Cong. C.S.A. Stat. 191 (1864); Mitchell to Robertson, Apr. 1, 1864, roll 14, microfilm M625, RG 45; Mallory, General Order, Feb. 24, 1865, file N474, roll 160, microfilm M474, RG 109.

5. Hasegawa, *Matchless Organization*, 4–5; Act of Feb. 26, 1861, ch. 17, Prov. Cong. C.S.A. Stat. 38 (1862).

6. Act of Mar. 6, 1861, ch 29, Prov. Cong. C.S.A. Stat 47 (1864); Act of Mar. 16, 1861, ch. 58, Prov. Cong. C.S.A. Stat. 70 (1864).

7. USND, *Instructions for the Government* (1857), 4,5; CSND, *Regulations*, 122–24; CSND, *Instructions for the Guidance*, 34–35. Although *flag officer* formally applied to an officer commanding a squadron, the title was also an honorary one for former squadron commanders. The term *commodore* was used in much the same way. Neither title was a formal CSN grade.

8. French Forrest to Green, Dec. 13, 1862, ZB file for Green, Navy Department Library.

9. Buchanan to Mallory, Dec. 29, 1862, ZB file for Minor, Navy Department Library.

10. Voucher for I.C. Dubose & Co., Dec. 23, 1862, roll 14, SF; Payrolls, July–Dec. 1863, Mobile, roll 16, MF; Pay table, CSND, *Register ... to January 1, 1864*, 55–56.

11. John K. Mitchell to Greenhow, Feb. 1, 1864, ZB file for Mitchell, Navy Department Library.

12. Callahan, *List of Officers*, 127; Muster and pay rolls, New Orleans, 1861, roll 169, MF; Muster and pay rolls, Richmond, 1862, roll 172, MF; Pay table, CSND, *Register... to January 1, 1864*, 55–56. A payroll showing Conrad's higher pay has not been found, but payroll entries for another fleet surgeon, James W.B. Greenhow, do show the $3,300 annual salary (Muster and pay rolls, Wilmington and CSS *Yadkin*, 1864, roll 165, MF).

13. Pay table, USND, *Register* (1861), 3; Hasegawa, "Officers' Promotions."

14. Bill S. 93, Sept. 22, 1862, entry 163, RG 109; *JCCSA*, 2:314. The bill's wording was published after the war, but its date of introduction, bill number, and fate were omitted (*ORN*, ser. 2, 2:57–58). Edwin G. Booth, who was a CSN assistant surgeon, strongly implied after the war that "first assistant surgeon" meant "passed assistant surgeon" (Booth to Superintendent of Naval War Records, Oct. 3, 1898, ZB file for Booth, Navy Department Library).

15. The broadside (Medical Officers of the Confederate States, Broadside, n.d., call no. 186-: 5, Broadside Collection, Virginia Museum of History and Culture) contained much of the wording that appeared in the bill. Full wording of the bill was published after the war with its title (Bill for the reorganization of the Medical Corps of the Confederate States Navy, *ORN*, ser. 2, 2:247–48) but without its date of introduction, bill number, or fate. *JCCSA* identifies a bill with the identical title as S. 20, which was introduced on January 28, 1863 (*JCCSA*, 3:37).

16. Act of Mar. 16, 1861, ch. 58, Prov. Cong. C.S.A. Stat. 70 (1864).

17. Bill for the reorganization of the Medical Corps of the Confederate States Navy, *ORN*, ser. 2, 2:247–48.

18. Bill for the reorganization of the

Notes—Chapter 5

Medical Corps of the Confederate States Navy, *ORN*, ser. 2, 2:247–48; Act of Feb. 21, 1861, ch. 49, § 3, 12 Stat. 147, 150 (1863); Act of Aug. 3, 1861, ch. 42, § 21–23, 12 Stat. 287, 290 (1863); Act of Dec. 31, 1861, ch. 1, § 1–3, 12 Stat. 329 (1863); USND, *Register* (1862), 24–26. In the postwar printing of the CSN bill, Mallory's addition nonsensically reads, "The service performed in the United States Navy by medical officers who have resigned therefrom, and are noncommissioned in the Confederate States Navy, shall be considered as having been performed under their present commissions." A handwritten version of the bill clarifies the meaning by showing "now commissioned" in place of "noncommissioned" (Bill for the reorganization of the Medical Corps of the Confederate States Navy, roll 15, SF).

19. Bill for the reorganization of the Medical Corps of the Confederate States Navy, *ORN*, ser. 2, 2:247–48; *JCCSA*, 3:164.

20. *JCCSA*, 3:31, 171.

21. *JCCSA*, 3:100, 164, 216, 220, 224–25, 231, 295–96, 370, 384; 6:67, 98, 120, 131–35, 295–96, 297, 449–51. Introduction of identical Senate and House bills was evidently one strategy for enhancing the likelihood of the legislation's passage. Part of the plan for Senate bill S. 93, introduced in September 1862, was to propose the same bill in the House "in view of saving trouble to the two committees & hope it will receive the approval & action of both houses" (Bill S. 93, Sept. 22, 1862, entry 163, RG 109).

22. *JCCSA*, 3:577; 4:12; 6:759; 7:82; M Mason to A.G. Brown, May 2, 1864, *ORN*, ser. 2, 2:648–50; H.R. 104, p. 29, vol. 19, ch. 7, RG 109.

23. Bill S. 189, Jan. 16, 1864, and bill S. 2, May 4, 1864, entry 163, RG 109.

24. Hasegawa, "Officers' Promotions"; S.S. Lee to Mallory, Oct. 31, 1864, *ORN*, ser. 2, 2:753–55.

25. CSND, *Register ... to January 1, 1864*, 12–17, 43–44; Gibbes and Morfit promotion nominations, Nov. 10, 1864, and confirmations, Nov. 28, 1864, *JCCSA*, 4:264, 296. Although Gibbes and Morfit were not promoted to passed assistant surgeon in the PNCS until November 1864, Gibbes performed satisfactorily on his surgeon examination in May 1864 and was told that his promotion to passed assistant surgeon would be effective as soon as the examining board adjourned. He started getting paid as a passed assistant surgeon no later than October 1, 1864 (Gibbes diary, May 9, 1864; Muster and pay rolls, 1864, Charleston Station, roll 166, MF). Morfit also seems to have performed satisfactorily at the same examining session, finished his examination on June 27, 1864, and started signing himself as a passed assistant surgeon no later than September 1864 (John K. Mitchell to Morfit, Apr. 12, 1864, roll 16, and voucher for W.H. Lippett, Sept. 8, 1864, roll 15, SF).

Chapter 5

1. Holden, "Hospital Corps"; G.R.B. Horner, *Diseases and Injuries of Seamen*, 14–16; USND, *Instructions for the Government* (1857), 8.

2. E. Cutbush, George Davis, Samuel R. Marshall, and Thomas Ewell. Report on Naval Hospitals, Mar. 16, 1812. *Annals of Congress*, 12th Cong., 1st sess., appendix, 2150–56; "Hospital Corps"; USND, *Register* (1860), 9; Isaac Toucey, *Report of the Secretary of the Navy*, Dec. 1, 1860, S. Exec. Doc. 1, 36th Cong., 2nd sess., 75–82 (1860).

3. CSND, *Instructions for the Guidance*, 6; Muster and pay rolls, New Orleans Station, 1861, roll 169, MF; CSND, *Register ... to January 1, 1863*, 29; CSND, *Register ... to January 1, 1864*, 58; Voucher for Minor, Dec. 6, 1861, roll 23, SF; Advertisement, *Daily Picayune* (New Orleans), Nov. 3, 1861, 3.

4. Muster and pay rolls, 1863, Richmond, VA, roll 172, MF; Payrolls, 1864, Savannah Station, roll 171, MF; Muster and pay rolls, 1862 and 1864, Charleston Station, roll 166, MF; Payrolls, Charleston, SC, entry 652, RG 45; Voucher for Spikes, Oct. 21, 1864, roll 15, SF.

5. CSND, *Instructions for the Guid-*

Notes—Chapter 6

ance, 6; USND, *Instruction for the Government* (1857); Muster and pay rolls, CSS *Dalman*, 1863, roll 16, MF; Muster and pay rolls, CSS *Virginia*, 1862, and Drewry's Bluff, 1863 and 1864, roll 172, MF; Muster and pay rolls, Warrington, FL, 1862, and payrolls, Warrington, FL, 1862, roll 165, MF.

6. CSND, *Regulations*, 30.

7. Advertisement, *Mobile Advertiser and Register*, Mar. 25, 1862, 2; Muster and pay rolls, CSS *Morgan*, 1862, roll 167, MF; Reports of the sick, 4th qtr., 1862, and 1st qtr., 1863, Medical Journal, CSS *Atlanta*, Confederate States of America: Medical Records, McCain Library and Archives; James Townsend, Report of the Master of Arms, June 19, 1863, *ORN*, ser. 1, 14:267–68; H.W. Wessells, extract of Special Orders no. 37, Office of Commissary General of Prisoners, Dec. 16, 1864, roll 44, SF.

8. Mallory, cost estimates, Mar. 12, 1861, entry 160, RG 109; Mallory to D.B. Conrad, Oct. 25, 1864, *OR*, ser. 2, 7:1086; Muster and pay rolls, Mobile, AL, 1862, roll 16, MF. Civilian hospital stewards working at land-based hospitals were unlikely to be taken prisoner, but Secretary Mallory was probably allowing for the possibility that the title of hospital steward could be applied to naval personnel.

9. Benedict, receipt, Dec. 4, 1861, microfilm roll 22, M331, RG 109; Hollins to Benedict, Dec. 18, 1861, and Minor to Steinriede, Dec. 10, 1861, ZB files for Benedict and Steinriede, Navy Department Library; Minor to Benedict, Dec. 30, 1861, Minor to Post, Jan. 31, 1862, Minor to Pelaez, Feb. 12, 1862, and Minor to Parker, Feb. 22, 1862, roll 20, SF. Steinriede used his middle name, Joseph, as his first during the Civil War.

10. Shipping articles for Benedict (Nov. 20, 1861), Steinriede (Dec. 11, 1861), Post (Jan. 31, 1862), Pelaez (Feb. 12, 1862), and Parker (Feb. 22, 1862), New Orleans, roll 173, MF; Muster and pay rolls for Benedict, Steinriede, Post, Pelaez, Parker, and Smith, New Orleans, roll 169, MF; Advertisement, *Daily Picayune* (New Orleans), Sept. 11, 1861, 1.

Chapter 6

1. J.D. Johnston to G. Floyd Johnston, Oct. 19, 1861, roll 19, SF; Vouchers for G. Floyd Johnston, Dec. 1861 and Mar. 1862, roll 14, SF; Voucher for G. Floyd Johnston, Apr. 19, 1862, ZB file for G. Floyd Johnston, Navy Department Library.

2. Vouchers for Hill, Dec. 11, 1863, and Jan. 13, 1864, both in roll 16; May 12, 1864, roll 14; and July 10, 1864, roll 15, SF.

3. Ancient Mariner [pseud.], "The Confederate Navy," *Daily Picayune* (New Orleans), May 5, 1861, 6; "Sad Accident—Four Lives Lost," *New Orleans Daily Crescent*, May 25, 1861, 7; "The Escape of the Pirate Sumter from the Iroquois," *Boston Morning Journal*, Jan. 13, 1862, 2.

4. Voucher for Goodloe, Nov. 18, 1861, roll 14, SF; Compiled service record for Goodloe, roll 108, microfilm M331, RG 109.

5. Vouchers for Hasenburg, July 10, 1861, Herndon, Apr. 5, 1862, and Archer, Apr. 2, 1864, roll 15, SF; Voucher for Ancrum, Nov. 7, 1862, roll 17, SF.

6. Vouchers for Wakefield, Dec. 1, 1862, and Johnston, Nov. 12, 1862, roll 15, SF; Muster rolls and payrolls for CSS *Chattahoochee*, 3rd qtr. 1862, roll 165, MF.

7. Vouchers for Savannah Marine Hospital, May 1861–July 1863, roll 15, SF. All references in this book to CSS *Georgia* are for the floating battery rather than the commerce raider.

8. CSND, *Regulations*, 31; Bill for Hall, Sept. 29, 1862, roll 15, SF.

9. Sinclair to Jones, Dec. 17, 1861, roll 19, SF; Officers and crew, CSS *Seabird*, roll 45, SF; Paroles for Jones and Hays, roll 44, SF; Hollins to Hays, Sept. 13, 1861, roll 19, SF; Muster roll, CSS *Selma*, roll 17, SF; Muster rolls and payrolls, CSS *Selma*, roll 16, MF.

10. "The Arkansas Attacked by Two Yankee Rams and a Gunboat," *Eastern Clarion* (Paulding, MS), Aug. 1, 1862, 1; Read, "Reminiscences of the Confederate States Navy," 357.

11. Read, "Reminiscences of the Confederate States Navy," 357.

Notes—Chapter 7

12. "The Arkansas Attacked by Two Yankee Rams and a Gunboat," *Eastern Clarion* (Paulding, MS), Aug. 1, 1862, 1.

13. R.B. Pegram to Mallory and list of officers of CSS *Nashville*, Mar. 10, 1862, *ORN*, ser. 1, 1:745–49, 752; Semmes, *Memoirs of Service Afloat*, 417, 598; Waddell to McNulty, Oct. 18, 1864, roll 20, SF; Riley, "The Stars and Bars: Exploits in the Pacific after the War Was Over," *Atlanta Constitution*, Nov. 26, 1893, 3; "Dr. M'Nulty Dead," *Sun* (New York), June 15, 1897, 5. *Alabama* was built in Liverpool, England. Most of its crewmembers were British and enlisted immediately after the vessel was commissioned at sea off of the Azores (Sinclair, *Two Years on the Alabama*, 10–16).

14. Information Concerning the Prison Records of Certain Naval Officers of the Confederate States…, roll 44, SF.

Chapter 7

1. John M. Brooks to Catesby ap R. Jones, June 15, 1863, roll 39, SF.

2. CSND, *Register … to January 1, 1863*, 11; CSND, *Register … to January 1, 1864*, 13; Cornick to S.S. Anderson, Feb. 13, 1862, file C273, roll 10, microfilm M474, RG 109; CSND, *Regulations*, 31.

3. Gibbes diary, multiply entries.

4. CSND, *Register … to January 1, 1864*, 12–17, 43–44.

5. Invoice for Benj. S. Thiess and Pollard, May 23, 1861, roll 14, SF; Requisition, July 23, 1861, roll 15, SF; File for Carrington, microfilm roll 49, M331, RG 109; Carrington to Samuel Preston Moore, Mar. 5, 1862, file C370, roll 11, microfilm M474, RG 109; Special Orders no. 27, para. 6, Feb. 3, 1862, and Special Orders no. 55, para. 14, Mar. 10, 1862, vol. 8, ch. 1, RG 109; Payrolls, Richmond Naval Station, 4th qtr. 1862 and 1st and 2nd qtrs. 1862, roll 172, MF; Payroll for CSS *Baltic*, 1st qtr. 1863, roll 13, MF.

6. Special Orders no. 119, para. 12, Aug. 9, 1861, vol. 6, ch. 1, RG 109; Phillips to Wise, Sept. 18, 1861, General Orders no. 104, Wise's Legion, Sept. 24, 1861, and Wise to Davis, Mar. 18, 1862, roll 97, microfilm M331, RG 109.

7. File for D.S. Green, roll 111, microfilm M331, RG 109; Samuel Preston Moore to B.W. Green, Aug. 14, 1861, ZB file for Green, Navy Department Library; Files for Christian, roll 55, microfilm M331, RG 109, and roll 71, microfilm M347, RG 109; Voucher for John B. Moore, Nov. 1, 1861, roll 14, SF; "Tribute of Respect," *Richmond Whig and Public Advertiser*, Mar. 15, 1864, 4.

8. Multiple entries, Daniel B. Conrad Diaries, Library of Congress; Lynn, *Confederate Commando and Fleet Surgeon*, 40–64; Welles to Conrad, May 10, 1861; roll 390, MF; CSND, *Register … to January 1, 1863*, 10; File for Conrad, roll 373, microfilm M324, RG 109.

9. Lynn, *Confederate Commando and Fleet Surgeon*, 106–8.

10. Bohemian [pseud.]. "Our Own Correspondent," *Daily Dispatch* (Richmond), Oct. 25, 1861, 2; Payrolls, Richmond Naval Station, 1861, roll 172, MF.

11. Mallory to Galt, Sept. 26, 1864, ZB file for Galt, Navy Department Library.

12. Wells, *Confederate Navy*, 139–141; CSND, *Regulations*, 190–93; Roberts, "What is a 'Naval Station'?"

13. Voucher for John Fraser & Co., Jan. 29, 1863, voucher for Woodman & Bement, Oct. 1, 1861; voucher for I.C. Dubose & Co., Apr. 4, 1863, and voucher for John B. Moore, Dec. 3, 1861, roll 14, SF; Voucher for Morfit, Mar. 9, 1864, roll 15, SF; Mallory to Carrington, May 2, 1861, ZB file for Carrington, Navy Department Library. Carrington's service as surgeon of the yard at Pensacola probably followed Spotswood's departure from that facility.

14. Voucher for David S. Johnston, Sept. 30, 1863, roll 15, SF; Franklin Buchanan to Herrick, Nov. 6, 1863, Buchanan to Caire, June 25, 1864, and French Forrest to Read, Nov. 26, 1864, ZB files for Herrick, Caire, and Read, Navy Department Library.

15. CSND, *Regulations*, 191.

16. General Orders no. 1 (June 15, 1863), no. 2 (June 16, 1863) and no. 3 (June 19, 1863), Papers of Lewis Willis Minor, Albert and Shirley Small Special Collections Library.

Notes—Chapter 8

17. Welles, *Confederate Navy*, 138–141; Hunter to Lee, Sept. 12 and 20, 1864, and Lee to Hunter, Sept. 16, 1864, roll 18, SF.

18. Mitchell to Galt, Nov. 11 and 12, 1864, and Mitchell to Washington, Nov. 13, 1864, ZB files for Galt and Washington, Navy Department Library.

19. John K. Mitchell to Williamson, Mar. 2, 1864, and William W. Hunter to Williamson, Mar. 7, 1864, Mitchell to Lynah, Feb. 1 and Mar. 1, 1864, ZB files for Williamson and Lynah, Navy Department Library.

20. Voucher for Purcell, Ladd & Co., Feb. 10, 1863, roll 15, SF; John K. Mitchell to Harrison, May 18, 1864, *ORN*, ser. 1, 10:642–43; Voucher for W.G. Trott, July 1, 1864, roll 14, SF; Voucher for W.H. Lippitt, Apr. 8, 1864, roll 15, SF; Conrad, report of killed and wounded, Aug. 1864, *OR*, ser. 1, vol. 39, pt. 1, 445. According to the USND *Register of Officers of the Confederate States Navy* (1931, p. 135), Surgeon Minor served as both station and fleet surgeon at Mobile in 1864–65. This appears to be erroneous, because during most of that time, Surgeon Conrad was fleet surgeon there. There is no record of Minor having a PNCS appointment, without which he supposedly would have been ineligible for service afloat—and for the office of fleet surgeon—during that time.

21. "Drewry's Bluff," *Daily Dispatch* (Richmond), May 1, 1863, 1; "Drewry's Bluff," *Hillsborough (NC) Recorder*, Aug. 12, 1863, 3; "For Drewry's Bluff!" *Daily Dispatch* (Richmond), Dec. 11, 1862, 2; Muster and pay rolls, Drewry's Bluff, roll 172, MF; CSND, *Register ... to January 1, 1863*; CSND, *Register ... to January 1, 1864*; Southerner [pseud.], "The Chickahominy Battle-fields," *Flag of Our Union* (Boston), Oct. 20, 1866, 659; "Editorial Correspondence of the Courier," *Charleston Tri-Weekly Courier*, Nov. 15, 1862, 2; Requisition for ambulance, May 20, 1862, roll 15, SF; John K. Mitchell to S.S. Lee, Oct. 5, 1864, and Mitchell to Lee, Oct. 16, *ORN*, ser. 1, 10:772–73, 785–86; Mitchell to Lee, Nov. 4, 1864, *ORN*, ser. 1, 11:753.

22. Gibbes diary, May 9 and 18, 1864.

23. Mallory to Garnett, Nov. 20, 1861, ZB file for Garnett, Navy Department Library.

24. Lamb, "Defense of Fort Fisher"; "List of Commissioned Officers," *Daily North Carolinian* (Wilmington), Jan. 30, 1865, 3; Information concerning the prison records of certain Naval Officers of the Confederate States, roll 44, SF; D.H. Hill, *North Carolina*, 489–90; S.S. Lee to Hicks, Nov. 1, 1864, ZB file for Hicks, Navy Department Library.

25. Becker, "Fort Fisher and Wilmington"; Lamb, "Defense of Fort Fisher."

26. Theophilus H. Holmes to Samuel Cooper, Nov. 25, 1862, *OR*, ser. 1, 13:927–28; David D. Porter to Gideon Welles, Jan. 16, 1863, *ORN*, ser. 1, 24:154; Porter to Welles, Jan. 12, 1863, *ORN*, ser. 1, 24:116–17; Porter to Wells, Jan. 17, 1863, USND, *Report of the Secretary of the Navy* (Dec. 1863), 415.

27. Waterman, "Notable Events of the Civil War."

28. D.E. Twiggs to Leroy P. Walker, July 12, 1861, *ORN*, ser. 1, 16:581–82; Warley to Edward Higgins, July 10, 1861, *OR*, ser. 1, vol. 53:708–10; "The Ship Island Engagement," *Daily Dispatch* (Richmond), July 23, 1861, 3; "Official Report of the Ship Island Expedition," *Charleston Daily Courier*, July 17, 1861, 1.

29. Dunnington to Thomas C. Hindman, June 21, 1862, *OR*, ser. 1, 13:929–31.

30. Sinclair, *Two Years on the Alabama*, 314–16; Kell, "Cruise and Combats of the 'Alabama.'"

31. Duncan N. Ingraham to John Grimball, May 11, 1863, roll 414, microfilm M625, RG 45; Abstract log of CSS *Florida*, Sept. 17, 1863–Mar. 31, 1864, *ORN*, ser. 1, 2:680–83; James D. Bulloch to George S. Shryock, Jan. 10, 1865, *ORN*, ser. 1, 3:729 30; Officers of CSS *Stonewall*, roll 18, SF; Diary from 1863 to 1865 for Captain S. Barron, CS Navy, *ORN*, ser. 2, 2:816–20.

Chapter 8

1. G.R.B. Horner, *Diseases and Injuries of Seamen*, 13; CSND, *Regulations*, 3;

Notes—Chapter 8

Spotswood to S.R. Mallory, Apr. 29, 1864, *ORN*, ser. 2, 2:647.

2. Mitchell to S.S. Lee, May 28 and 29, 1864, ZB files for Washington and Addison, Navy Department Library.

3. Muster and pay rolls, CSS *Palmetto State*, 1864, roll 166, MF. Freeman was promoted from assistant surgeon to passed assistant surgeon in February 1863.

4. CSND, *Regulations*, 121–28; John K. Mitchell to Mallory, June 27, 1864, *ORN*, ser. 1, 10:710–11.

5. G.R.B. Horner, *Diseases and Injuries of Seamen*, 52–53; J.N. Maffitt to Mallory, July 27, 1863, *ORN*, ser. 1, 2: 652–54.

6. CSND, *Instructions for the Guidance*.

7. Gibbes diary, May 25, 1863.

8. G.R.B. Horner, *Diseases and Injuries of Seamen*, 13–14, 45–50.

9. G.R.B. Horner, *Diseases and Injuries of Seamen*, 11–12.

10. G.R.B. Horner, *Diseases and Injuries of Seamen*, 13–14, 45–50; Wilson, *Naval Hygiene*, 13–14.

11. Medical journal, CSS *General Polk*, Confederate States of America: Medical Records, McCain Library and Archives; Medical journal, CSS *Gaines*, roll 15, SF.

12. Medical journal, CSS *Gaines*, roll 15, SF.

13. Medical journal, CSS *Gaines*, roll 15, SF; Abstract of quarterly reports, *ORN*, ser. 2, 2:562. The same patient could be admitted more than once, so the number of admissions was generally larger than the number of individual patients.

14. Medical journal, CSS *Gaines*, roll 15, SF.

15. Medical journal, CSS *Gaines*, roll 15, SF; USND, *Dictionary of American Naval Fighting Ships*, vol. 2, 522; Buchanan to Mallory, Aug. 13, 1864, file N355, roll 77, microfilm M474, RG 109; Mitchell to George E. Pickett, August 10, 1864, *ORN*, ser. 1, 10:731.

16. Mitchell to S.S. Lee, November 4, 1864, *ORN*, ser. 1, 11:753; William W. Hunter to Lee, September 20, 1864, roll 18, SF; Ewart obituary, *Charleston Daily Courier*, Oct. 14, 1864, 2.

17. CSND, *Ordnance Instructions*, 16, 32; Ruschenberger, Review, 415–16; Read, "Reminiscences of the Confederate States Navy," 356; Medical journal, CSS *General Polk*, Mar. 6, 1862, Confederate States of America: Medical Records, McCain Library and Archives.

18. Ruschenberger, Review, 415–16; CSND, *Ordnance Instructions*, 16, 32; Wilson, *Naval Hygiene*, 150; Jim Dan Hill, *Civil War Sketchbook*, 48–49, 55; Read, "Reminiscences of the Confederate States Navy," 353.

19. CSND, *Ordnance Instructions*, 93.

20. Parker, *Recollections of a Naval Officer*, 237–38.

21. CSND, *Ordnance Instructions*, 8; Conrad, "Capture of the C.S. Ram Tennessee."

22. Conrad, "Capture of the C.S. Ram Tennessee"; Buchanan to S.R. Aug. 25, 1864, *ORN*, ser. 1, 21:576–79.

23. Iglehart to J.W. Bennett, Aug. 9, 1864, *ORN*, ser. 1, 21:590–91; Bennett to Mallory, Aug. 8, 1864, *ORN*, ser. 1, 21: 588–90.

24. Rochard, "Surgical Services," May 31, 1862, 300; Bollet, "Amputations"; G.R.B. Horner, *Diseases and Injuries of Seamen*, 70–71, 214–15, 219–20, 222–23.

25. Buchanan to Mallory, Mar. 27, 1862, *ORN*, ser. 1, 7:44–49; Read to W.C. Whittle, May 1, 1862, *ORN*, ser. 1, 18:332–33; Pierson to Gideon Welles, Sept. 10, 1864, *ORN*, ser. 1, 15:481–83.

26. Medical journal, CSS *General Polk*, Jan 2, 1862, and medical journal, CSS *Atlanta*, Feb. 14 and June 4, 1863, Confederate States of America: Medical Records, McCain Library and Archives.

27. "Surgeon of the Alabama"; Sinclair, *Two Years on the Alabama*, 316–17; Kell, "Cruise and Combats of the 'Alabama.'"

28. Jackstay [pseud.], "Wreck of the C.S.S. Chattahoochee," *Daily Sun* (Columbus, GA), June 2, 1863, 2; Justice [pseud.], "The 'Chattahoochee' Disaster," *Daily Sun* (Columbus, GA), June 7, 1863; Thomas Moreno to D.B. Harris, May 26 and 28, 1863, *OR*, ser. 1,15:954;

Notes—Chapter 9

A. McLaughlin to Catesby ap. R. Jones, June 1 and 15, 1863, *ORN*, ser. 1, 17:868, 869–71; Voucher for Ford, June 2, 1863, roll 15, SF; Chenoweth and Mock, "Hurricane 'Amanda.'"

29. Medical journal, CSS *Atlanta*, Apr. 1, 1863, Confederate States of America: Medical Records, McCain Library and Archives; Medical journal, CSS *Gaines*, June 28, Sept. 3, Sept. 17, Oct. 7, Nov. 11, and Dec. 14, 1862, and May 23, May 30, and July 3, 1863, roll 15, SF; Hasegawa, "Piscine Perils."

30. Gibbes diary, Feb. 23, 1863.

31. C.A. Boutelle to Francis A. Roe, May 6, 1864, roll 43, SF; Moore, *Rebellion Record*, documents section, 35; D.G. Farragut to Gideon Welles, Aug. 22 1864, *ORN*, ser. 1, 21:609–10; N. Collins to Welles, Oct. 31, 1864, *ORN*, ser. 1, 3:255–56; James Townsend, report, June 19, 1863, *ORN*, ser. 1, 14:267–68; John M. Brown to William Whelan, July 23, 1864, *ORN*, ser. 1, 3:69–71; D.D. Porter to Welles, May 2, 1862, *ORN*, ser. 1, 18:439–40; List of officers and crew of the late CS Str. *Seabird*, and List of officers and men, late of the Confederate Steamer *Oconee*, and now prisoners on board the USS *Madgie*, roll 44, SF; "The Loss of the Atlanta," *Charleston Daily Courier*, Dec. 29, 1863, 1; "Extracts from My 'Journal,' while a Prisoner in Port Royal Bay, S.C.," *Charleston Daily Courier*, Jan. 12, 1864, 1, and Jan. 13, 1864, 1; Gibbes diary, June 16, 1863 [Jan. 1864?], and Dec. 29, 1863.

32. O'Brien and Diefendorf, *General Orders*, 261; Information concerning the prison records of certain Naval Officers of the Confederate States, roll 44, SF; Farragut to Welles, Aug. 22, 1864, *ORN*, ser. 1, 21:609–10; Farragut to C.C. Dwight, Nov. 2, 1864, *ORN*, ser. 2, 7: 1085–86; Mallory to Conrad, Oct. 25, 1864, *ORN*, ser. 2, 7:1086. USN prisoners in the custody of the CSN were to be turned over to the Confederate army (Act of May 2, 1861, ch. 54, Prov. Cong. C.S.A. Stat. 154 [1864]).

33. Goldsborough to Welles, Feb. 14, 1862, and Goldsborough to Benjamin Huger, Feb. 12 and 14, 1862, in USND, *Report of the Secretary of the Navy* (Dec. 1862), 83–85; Conrad, "Capture of the C.S. Ram Tennessee"; "From Pensacola," *Daily Sun* (Columbus, GA), Sept. 11, 1864, 2; Farragut to C.C. Dwight, Nov. 2, 1864, *ORN*, ser. 2, 7:1085–86; Information concerning the prison records of certain Naval Officers of the Confederate States, roll 44, SF.

34. McLain, "Military Prison at Fort Warren"; Bowles, "The Ship Tennessee," *Times* (Richmond), Oct. 5, 1893, 2.

Chapter 9

1. England, "American Manufacture of Quinine Sulphate"; Cole, "Manufacture and Consumption"; Freedley, *Philadelphia and Its Manufactures*, 207–8.

2. Freedley, *Leading Pursuits*, 113–35; Zeilin, "Drug Business."

3. "Commercial Dependence of the South on the North"; Wise, *Lifeline of the Confederacy*, 12; C.A. Wood and Nichols, "Annual Report on Drugs"; C.A. Wood and Nichols, "Review of the Drug Trade"; Act of Feb. 18, 1861, ch. 3, § 2, Prov. Cong. C.S.A. Stat. 28 (1864); Act of Feb. 26, 1861, ch. 16, Prov. Cong. C.S.A. Stat. 38 (1864).

4. Nichols, "Review of the New York Markets"; Lincoln, Proclamations of Apr. 19 and 27, 1861, *OR*, ser. 3, 1:89–90, 122; "What Articles are Contraband of War," *Boston Evening Transcript*, May 16, 1861, 4.

5. Carney et al., "Report on Home Adulterations."

6. William Whelan to James C. Dobbin, Oct. 28, 1854, H.R. Exec. Doc. 33rd Cong., 2nd sess., 577–80 (1854); Whelan to Dobbin, Oct. 29, 1855; S. Exec. Doc. 1, 34th Cong., 1st sess., 278–84 (1855); USND, *Instructions for the Government* (1857), 3.

7. Hasegawa, *Matchless Organization*, 59–68.

8. Brewer et al., "Report of the Committee on the Drug Market," 270.

9. USND, *Instructions for the Government* (1857); CSND, *Instructions for the Guidance*; United States War Department, *Revised Regulations*, 292–301;

Notes—Chapter 9

Vouchers for Dawson & Blackman, Feb. 13 and Apr. 27, 1863, roll 14, SF.

10. CSND, *Instructions for the Guidance*, 3–4; Voucher for E.B. Wheelock, May 3, 1861, and voucher for Theiss & Pollard, May 23, 1861, roll 14, SF.

11. Vouchers for James Syme, May 9, 1861, A.A. Solomons, June 13, 1861, B. & J. Abrams, Nov. 28, 1861, Pharmacie Podevin, Dec. 14, 1863, and Jan. 11, 1864, J.B. Baillière, Jan. 5, 1864, A.A. Solomons, Dec. 31, 1861, and Urquhart & Chapman, Mar. 19, 1864, roll 14, SF; Voucher for John B. Hall & Sons, Aug. 3, 1861, 15, SF.

12. Requisitions, May 20 and Dec. 29, 1862, roll 15, SF; Vouchers for Lining, Oct. 3, 1862, Nov. 1, 1862, and May 22, 1863, roll 14, SF; W.J. Addison to Smith, Sept. 7, 1862, and receipt for supplies issued by Potts to Addison, Sept. 14, 1862, roll 2, microfilm M331, RG 109.

13. Spotswood to Mallory, Mar. 11, 1862, with endorsements, file P203, roll 39, microfilm M474, RG 109; Special Orders no. 59, para. 25, Mar. 14, 1862, vol. 8, ch. 1, RG 109.

14. Voucher for F.E. Ward, Sept. 25, 1862, roll 15, SF; Voucher for Richard Hall, Dec. 5, 1862, roll 14, SF; Coski, *Capital Navy*, 20; Voucher for William Ritter, May 11, 1863, roll 14, SF; Voucher, Dec. 4, 1862, ZB file for Patton, Navy Department Library; Spotswood to Mallory, Nov. 30, 1863, *ORN*, ser. 2, 2:559–61.

15. Spotswood to Mallory, Nov. 30, 1863, *ORN*, ser. 2, 2:559–61.

16. Vouchers for Purcell, Ladd & Co., Feb. 10, May 2, and May 25, 1863, roll 15, SF; Muster and pay roll, CSS *Stono*, June 1863, roll 18, MF; Voucher for Lecky, May 1863, and voucher for J.W. Thomas Jr., June 19, 1863, roll 15, SF.

17. Dowden to George W. Randolph, Mar. 27, 1862, roll 256, microfilm M346, RG 109; Vouchers for Dowden, Nov. 10 and Dec. 10, 1863, roll 15, SF; Spotswood to Mallory, Nov. 1, 1864, *ORN*, ser. 2, 2: 758–62.

18. Hays to DeBree Jr., May 13, 1863, and John K. Mitchell to Cook, Apr. 29, 1864, ZB files for DeBree Jr., and Cook, Navy Department Library.

19. Spotswood to Mallory, Nov. 30, 1863, and Nov. 1, 1864, *ORN*, ser. 2, 2:559–61, 758–62; Mallory to John Taylor Wood, July 23, 1864, roll 413, microfilm M625, RG 45; Hasegawa and Hambrecht, "Confederate Medical Laboratories."

20. Confederate States Army Medical Department, *General Directions*; Confederate States Army Medical Department, *Standard Supply Table of the Indigenous Remedies*; Porcher, *Resources of Southern Fields and Forests*; Hasegawa, *Matchless Organization*, 77–82.

21. Vouchers for Purcell, Ladd & Co., Dec. 16, 1862, and June 3, 1863, for Lecky, May 25, 1863, and for Robertson, Oct. 1, 1863, roll 15, SF; Hasegawa, *Matchless Organization*, 77–82; Spotswood to Mallory, Nov. 30, 1863, *ORN*, ser. 2, 2: 559–63.

22. Spotswood to Mallory, Nov. 1, 1864, *ORN*, ser. 2, 2:758–60.

23. Hasegawa, *Matchless Organization*, 75–77; Vouchers for Koch, Aug. 16, 1862, and July 10, 1864, roll 14, SF, and Apr. 25, 1864, roll 558, microfilm M346, RG 109; Voucher for Harley, July 2, 1864, roll 15, SF.

24. Advertisement, *Charleston Daily Courier*, Sept. 26, 1862, 2.

25. Voucher for James Syme, May 9, 1861, roll 14, SF; Voucher for J.W. Thomas, June 19, 1863, and voucher for John B. Moore, June 25, 1863, roll 15, SF; Voucher for William Henry Belden, Sept. 30, 1863, roll 14, SF; Voucher for E. & T. Sill, Nov. 8, 1864, and vouchers for Thomas H. Morris, June 1 and Aug. 12, 1864, roll 15, SF; Weidenmier, "Turning Points."

26. Spotswood to Mallory, Nov. 1, 1864, *ORN*, ser. 2, 2:758–62; Wise, *Lifeline of the Confederacy*, 241, 267–68, 272–73; Voucher for Wysham, Mar. 26, 1864, voucher for J.C. Dubose, Sept. 30, 1864, and Wysham to Ware, May 7, 1864, roll 14, SF; Invoice for *Denbigh*, June 1, 1864, roll 45, SF; Jonathan L. Carter to Page, Feb. 24, 1864, roll 15, SF.

27. Act of Aug. 29, 1842, ch. 267, 5 Stat. 546 (1856); Act of Aug 3, 1848, ch. 121, § 5, 9 Stat. 266, 271 (1862); Rations—Provisional Navy of the Confederate States, n.d., roll 51, SF; CSND, *Instructions for*

Notes—Chapter 10

the *Guidance*, 8–11; George B. Wood and Bache, *Dispensatory*, 62–67. The CSN emulated the USN regarding rations and commutation rates.

28. Voucher for R.W. Abrams & Co., June 22, 1861, expenditure documents, July 3, Aug. 23, and Nov. 1, 1861, roll 51, SF; DeBree Sr., to Mallory, Nov. 14, 1863, *ORN*, ser. 2, 2:552–57; John K. Mitchell, general order, Nov. 28, 1863; *ORN*, ser. 1, 15:696–97.

29. Voucher for Purcell, Ladd & Co., Nov. 26, 1861, voucher for John B. Moore, Aug. 1, 1862, voucher for A.A. Solomons & Co., Jan. 1, 1864, and voucher for W.H. Peterson, July 1, 1864, roll 15, SF.

30. Burton N. Harrison, letter to the editor, *Daily Richmond Enquirer*, Feb. 26, 1864, 4; Davis to Mallory, Mar. 7, 1864, OR, ser. 4, vol. 3, pt. 2, 879–80; Act of June 14, 1864, ch. 41, C.S.A. Stat. 271 (1864).

Chapter 10

1. Register of Confederate Naval Patients in the C.S. Hospital Ship "St. Philip" at New Orleans, Louisiana, and Register of Confederate Naval Patients in the Charity Hospital at New Orleans, Louisiana, Papers of Lewis Willis Minor, Albert and Shirley Small Special Collections Library; "Meeting of the Ladies," *Daily Sun* (Columbus, GA), May 22, 1861, 3; "Soldier's Home," *Daily Sun* (Columbus, GA), May 15, 1862, 3; Confederated Southern Memorial Association, *History of the Confederate Memorial Associations*, 116–17; Catesby ap R. Jones to Ford, Nov. 27, 1862, ZB file for Jones, Navy Department Library; Voucher for Ford, May 22, 1863, roll 14, SF; Voucher for Ford, June 2, 1863, roll 15, SF; A. McLaughlin to Jones, June 15, 1863, *ORN*, ser. 1, 17:869–71; "Report of the 'Soldiers' Friend Society' for the Month of June," *Daily Sun* (Columbus, GA), July 12, 1862, 2; "Report of Soldier's Friend Society for July, 1862," *Daily Sun* (Columbus, GA), Aug. 6, 1862, 1; Compiled service record for Wingfield, roll 271, and for Colzey, roll 60, microfilm M331, RG 109.

2. W. Whelan to Gideon Welles, Oct. 23, 1863, H.R. Exec. Doc. 1, 38th Cong., 1st sess., 1059 (1863); John F. Hammond, "Medical Topography and Diseases of Barrancas Barracks." S. Exec. Doc. 96, 34th Cong., 1st sess., 325–29 (1856); USND, *Register* (1861); Lyles to Victor M. Randolph, Jan. 21, 25, and 28, 1861, roll 30, SF. During the Civil War, the building housing the Pensacola Marine Hospital (originally under the charge of the U.S. Treasury Department) appears to have been located at the mouth of Bayou Texar, by the eastern edge of Pensacola (*Daily Dispatch* [Richmond], June 24, 1854, 4).

3. Hacklander, list of sick, Feb. 9, 1861, Hacklander to Randolph, Feb. 11, 1861, and Bishop to Randolph, Jan. 14, 1861, roll 30, SF; Mallory, estimates, Mar. 12, 1861, entry 160, RG 109; Payrolls, 1861 and 1862, rolls 18 and 165, MF. Grafton's pay entry for July 1861 was for 112 days, so it may have covered duty back to April 1861.

4. Braxton Bragg to Samuel Jones, Feb. 27, 1862, OR, ser. 1, 6:835–36; Jones to John H. Forney, May 14, 1862, *ORN*, ser. 1, 18:482–44; David D. Porter to Gideon Welles, May 10, 1862, *ORN*, ser. 1, 18: 478–80; W. Whelan to Gideon Welles, Oct. 23, 1863, H.R. Exec. Doc. 1, 38th Cong., 1st sess., 1059 (1863).

5. W. Whelan to Gideon Welles, Oct. 23, 1863, H.R. Exec. Doc. 1, 38th Cong., 1st sess., 1059 (1863); D.G. Farragut to N.P. Banks, Jan. 27, 1863 [1864], *ORN*, ser. 1, 21:62; Whelan to Welles, Nov. 4, 1864, H.R. Exec. Doc. 1, 38th Cong., 2nd. sess., 1181 (1864); Buchanan to Mallory, Aug. 25, 1864, *ORN*, ser. 1, 21:576–78; Conrad, "Capture of the C.S. Ram Tennessee"; Sternberg, "Fort Barrancas, Florida"; Wales, *Sanitary and Statistical Report*, 434.

6. McCauley to Gideon Welles, April 25, 1861, *ORN*, ser. 1, 4:288–89; William H. Peters to John Letcher, Oct. 19, 1861, *ORN*, ser. 2, 2:107–12; William Whelan to Wells, Nov. 11, 1861, S. Comm. Rep. 37, 37th Cong., 2nd sess., 88 (1862). Like the hospital, the navy yard was referred to as being at Norfolk, Gosport, and Portsmouth.

Notes—Chapter 10

7. Minor to Gideon Welles, Apr. 18, 1861, roll 389, MF; Mason to Welles, Apr. 17, 1861, Sinclair to Welles, Apr. 23, 1861, Wysham to Welles, Apr. 25, 1861, Williamson to Welles, May 2, 1861, and Minor to Welles, May 13, 1861, roll 390, MF; John Letcher, Proclamation of June 6, 1861, *Richmond Daily Whig*, June 7, 1861, 2; French Forrest to T.T. Hunter, May 10, 1861, *ORN*, ser. 1, 4:407–8. Although Sinclair tendered his resignation from Philadelphia, he was reportedly attached to the Norfolk station at the time of its abandonment (H. Paulding to Welles, Apr. 23, 1861, *ORN*, ser. 1, 4:289–92).

8. Muster and pay rolls, New Orleans, 3rd qtr. 1862, roll 169, MF; Vouchers for H.L. Pauli and for M.A. and C.A. Santos, Sept. 30, 1861, roll 14, SF; Death notice, *Richmond Whig and Public Advertiser*, Jan. 24, 1862, 1; Paymaster account for Blacknall, Jan. 31, 1862, roll 16, SF; Franklin Buchanan to Cornick, Jan. 23, 1862, ZB file for Cornick, Navy Department Library; Cornick to S.S. Anderson, Feb. 13, 1862, with endorsement by Huger, file C273, roll 10, microfilm M474, RG 109.

9. Special Orders no. 56, para. 5, Mar. 11, 1862, vol. 8, ch. 1, RG 109; Porcher to Jenny, Mar. 15, 1862, Francis Peyre Porcher Papers, Waring Historical Library; Buchanan to Mallory, Mar. 27, 1862, *ORN*, ser. 1, 7:44–49; Thomas R. Ware to John Johnson, Mar. 18 and 31, 1862, roll 15, SF.

10. John Taylor Wood, "First Fight of Iron-Clads"; W. Whelan to Gideon Welles, Nov. 4, 1864, H.R. Exec. Doc. 1, 38th Cong., 2nd, sess., 1181 (1864); Whelan to Welles, Oct. 23, 1863, H.R. Exec. Doc. 1, 38th Cong., 1st sess., 1059 (1863).

11. Multiple vouchers for Ritter, rolls 14 and 43, SF; *Butters' Richmond Directory*, 138; *JCCSA*, 7:557.

12. Spotswood, notice, *Daily Dispatch* (Richmond), May 19, 1862, 3; Minor, advertisements, *Daily Dispatch* (Richmond), June 3 and 17, 1862, 3; Vouchers for G. & A. Bergamin, July 12, 1862, and for M.T. Clarke, Mar. 28, 1863, roll 14, SF; Voucher for Purcell, Ladd & Co., May 10, 1862, and for R.C. Howe, June 3, 1862, roll 15, SF.

13. CSND, *Register ... to January 1, 1863*, 10–11; CSND, *Register ... to January 1, 1864*, 12–17, 43–44; Muster and pay rolls, Richmond Naval Hospital, roll 172, MF; Harrison to DeBree Jr., Jan. 1, Mar. 4, May 6, June 1, June 3, and June 15, 1863, and Jan. 1, 1864, roll 15, SF; Voucher for Thomas J. Bagby, June 26, 1862, and vouchers for Hall, June 1, June 30, Aug. 1, and Sept. 30, 1863, roll 14, SF.

14. CSN patients in army hospitals, roll 1, microfilm M260, RG 109; Harrison to surgeon in charge, General Hospital No. 21, and Lindsay to unknown, Dec. 9, 1862, roll 15, SF; William A. Carrington, statistics of the variolous diseases, Jan. 16, 1863, vol. 416, ch. 6, RG 109.

15. News item, *Fayetteville (NC) Observer*, July 14, 1862, 1; "Died," *Daily Dispatch* (Richmond), Aug. 6, 1862, 2; J.P. Ralls, Committee Report, Apr. 21, 1862, *JCCSA*, 5:588–89; Calcutt, *Richmond's Wartime Hospitals*, 58–61.

16. Abstract of sick, *ORN*, ser. 2, 2:562–63, 761; Thomas R. Rootes (for John K. Mitchell) to S.S. Lee, Aug. 22, 1864, *ORN*, ser. 1, 10:734–35; Harrison to Joynes, Mar. 20, 1865, Sanger Historical Files, Tompkins–McCaw Library.

17. Muster and pay rolls, Mobile, AL, roll 16, MF; Advertisement, *Mobile Evening News*, Aug. 20, 1863, 2; Vouchers for Ross & Ketchum, Mar. 22 and June 30, 1864, roll 885, microfilm M346, RG 109, and Sept. 30, 1864, roll 14, SF; CSND, *Register ... to January 1, 1863*, 10–11; CSND, *Register ... to January 1, 1864*, 14–15, 44; Garnett, Booth, and Graves to Franklin Buchanan, Apr. 26, 1864, roll 16, SF. The first available payroll for the hospital is for the fourth quarter of 1862, but one nurse was paid for work starting July 1, 1862.

18. Muster and pay rolls, Mobile, roll 16, MF; Minor, notice, *Daily Dispatch* (Richmond), Oct. 3, 1862, 4; Pension application no. 19964 for Elizabeth A. McWilkie, fiche 5437, microfiche M1274, RG 15.

19. Voucher for Goodman, Sept. 30, 1864, and buildings used for Navy Depart-

Notes—Chapter 10

ment, roll 43, SF; J.E. Meire, advertisement, *Mobile Advertiser and Register*, Mar. 1, 1863, 2; Vouchers for Minor, Mar. 18 and June 1, 1864, roll 14, SF; Farrand to Minor, Aug. 16, 1864, roll 411, microfilm M625, RG 45.

20. Abstracts of sick, *ORN*, ser. 2, 2: 563, 761.

21. S.S. Lee to Booth, Nov. 1, 1864, with notations, ZB file for Booth, Navy Department Library; Muster and pay rolls, Mobile Station, roll 16, MF; Entries for Booth, Jan. 19 (p. 101) and Mar. 2, 1865 (p. 249), vol. 665, ch. 6, RG 109.

22. Voucher for Charles W. Boyd, Nov. 10, 1862, and Steinriede, requisition, Dec. 29, 1862, roll 15, SF; Voucher for Barksdale & McFarland, Oct.18, 1862, roll 14, SF.

23. Muster and pay rolls, Charleston Station, roll 166, MF; Vouchers for Pelzer, Jan. 12, 1864, roll 14, SF; Vouchers for Pelzer, May 12, 1864, and Oct. 6, 1864, roll 43, SF; "Soldiers' Directory of Public Offices," *Charleston Daily Courier*, Jan. 6, 1864, 2; CSND, *Register ... to January 1, 1864*, 43.

24. Muster and pay rolls, Charleston Station, roll 166, MF; Payrolls, Charleston, SC, entry 652, RG 45; Woodworth, *First Annual Report*, 8–9; News item, *Charleston Mercury*, Nov. 8, 1861 4; Voucher for Evans, Sept. 16, 1863, roll 14, SF; 1860 U.S. Census, District of Charleston, SC, population schedule, 4th ward, city of Charleston p. 325 (57 penned), dwelling 394, family 397, Evans family, roll 1216, microfilm M653, RG 29.

25. Abstracts of sick, *ORN*, ser. 2, 2: 562, 761.

26. Gibbes diary, Feb. 14–Apr. 14, 1865.

27. Multiple vouchers for medical care and rent, roll 15, SF; Lee and Agnew, *Historical Record*, 163; Sheehy and Wallace, *Savannah: Immortal City*, 12; S.M. Clark to S.P. Chase, Sept. 30, 1861, H.R. Exec. Doc., 37th Cong., 2nd sess., 97–112 (1861).

28. Multiple vouchers for Horace Morse, and vouchers for A.B. Clark, July 9 and Aug. 5, 1863, roll 14, SF; "Fire," *Daily Chronicle & Sentinel* (Augusta, GA) May 24, 1862, 1; "Fire in Savannah," *Wilmington (NC) Journal*, Nov. 26, 1863, 1; News item, *Weekly Chronicle & Sentinel* (Augusta, GA), Mar. 2, 1864, 3; Abstract of sick, *ORN*, ser. 2, 2:562.

29. Multiple vouchers for Elliott C. Johnson, Savannah Poor House Hospital, Savannah Hospital Association, and Savannah Gas Light Company, rolls 14, 42, and 43, SF.

30. Pierson to J.A. Dahlgren, Sept. 10, 1864, *ORN*, ser. 1, 15:481–88; CSND, *Register ... to January 1, 1864*, 16–17, 44; Payrolls, Savannah Naval Hospital, roll 171, MF; Billings, "Only Yesterday" (typescript), Luther Guiteau Billings Articles and Photographs, Library of Congress. Melton (*Best Station of Them All*, 308, 330) mentions a CSN hospital on Liberty Street in Savannah. This was probably the army's General Hospital No. 1, located at Oglethorpe Barracks on Liberty Street, which received CSN patients after the February 1864 Gibbons House fire. Oglethorpe Barracks also received wounded and unwounded USN prisoners from the captured *Water Witch* ("Capture of the Steamer Water Witch," *Weekly Intelligencer* [Fayetteville, NC], June 14, 1864, 2; A.D. Stover, correspondence, *Ellsworth (ME) American*, Nov. 25, 1864, 1).

31. Abstracts of sick, *ORN*, ser. 2, 2:562–63, 761; Payrolls, Savannah Naval Hospital, roll 171, MF.

32. "Great Conflagration," *Savannah Daily Herald*, Jan. 28, 1865, 2.

33. Commentary, *Wilmington (NC) Journal*, November 27 1862, 4; Vouchers for W.H. Hill, Dec. 11, 1863, and Jan. 13, 1863, roll 16, SF; "Hospital Directory," *Daily North Carolinian* (Wilmington), Dec. 30, 1864, 1; CSND, *Register ... to January 1, 1864*; Abstract, *ORN*, ser. 2, 2:761.

34. Charles K. Graham, report, Jan. 25, 1864, *OR*, ser. 1, 33:425–26; W.F. Lynch to W.H.C. Whiting, Mar. 2, 1864, *OR*, ser. 1, 33:1227; Multiple vouchers for Everitt, roll 43, SF; Spotswood to Mallory, Apr. 28, 1864, *ORN*, ser. 2, 2:647.

35. Voucher for J.J. Bloodgood, Sept. 12, 1861, roll 14, SF; CSND, *Register ... to*

Notes—Chapter 11

January 1, 1863, 10–13; Southerner, "The Chickahominy Battle-fields," *Flag of Our Union* (Boston), Oct. 20, 1866, 659. The *Flag of Our Union* article, which mentions the hospitals at Drewry's Bluff, was reprinted in 1906 and attributed to William S. Birgl ("Recollections of a Confederate," *Richmond Times Dispatch*, Aug. 12, 1906, 30).

36. Spotswood to Jeffery, June 9, 1862, ZB file for Jeffery, Navy Department Library.

37. "Surgeons Appalated for the Floating Battery," *New York Times*, March 12, 1861, 2; "The Hospital Attached to the Floating Battery in Charleston Harbor," *Frank Leslie's Illustrated Newspaper*, Mar. 30, 1861, 289–90.

38. "Letter from 'The Ancient Mariner,'" *New Orleans Weekly Crescent*, June 1, 1861, 6; Voucher for Woodman & Bement, Dec. 31, 1861, vouchers for Conrad, Nov. 25, 1861, and Apr. 29, 1862, and vouchers for B. & J. Abrams, Nov. 11 and 26, 1861, roll 14, SF; Whittle to Minor, Apr. 24, 1862, roll 410, microfilm M625, RG 45; Register of Confederate Naval Patients in the C.S. Hospital Ship "St. Philip" at New Orleans, Louisiana, and Register of Confederate Naval Patients in the Charity Hospital at New Orleans, Louisiana, Papers of Lewis Willis Minor, Albert and Shirley Small Special Collections Library.

39. A. Heiman to W.W. Mackall, Feb. 8, 1862, *ORN*, ser. 1, 22:564–69; Lloyd Tilghman to Samuel Cooper, Feb. 12, 1862, *ORN*, ser. 1, 22:553–62; J.P. McCown to G.T. Beauregard, Mar. 23, 1862, *ORN*, ser. 1, 22:742; "Latest from Island Ten," *Daily Picayune* (New Orleans), Apr. 8, 1862, 1; Voucher for William H. Davis, Oct. 31, 1861, roll 14, SF.

40. Gibbes diary, May 9, 1864; Scharf, *History of the Confederate States Navy*, 776; Herndon, "The Confederate States Naval Academy," 309–10.

Chapter 11

1. W.A.W. Spotswood to S.R. Mallory, Nov. 30, 1863, and Nov. 1, 1864, *ORN*, ser. 2, 2:559–63, 758–62.

2. Spotswood to Mallory, Nov. 30, 1863, and Nov. 1, 1864, *ORN*, ser. 2, 2: 559–63, 758–62.

3. Register of Confederate Naval Patients in the C.S. Hospital Ship "St. Philip" at New Orleans, Louisiana, and Register of Confederate Naval Patients in the Charity Hospital at New Orleans, Louisiana, Papers of Lewis Willis Minor, Albert and Shirley Small Special Collections Library; Medical journals, CSS *General Polk* and CSS *Atlanta*, Confederate States of America: Medical Records, McCain Library and Archives; Medical journal, CSS *Gaines*, roll 15, SF. Reported ages and countries of origin were sometimes inconsistent among patients admitted multiple times. The patients on CSS *Gaines* reportedly born in Manila may have been connected with a Filipino settlement near New Orleans. Passed Assistant Surgeon Charles E. Lining of CSS *Shenandoah* kept a journal of the vessel's cruise, but it has little medical content ("Journal of Charles E. Lining, C.S.S. Shenandoah").

4. G.R.B. Horner, *Diseases and Injuries of Seamen*, 9.

5. Andrew McIlwaine Bell, *Mosquito Soldiers*, 10–13; Wilson, *Naval Hygiene*, 162–67; CSND, *Instructions for the Guidance*, 24.

6. Spotswood to Mallory, Nov. 30, 1863, *ORN*, ser. 2, 2:559–61; Medical journal, CSS *Gaines*, roll. 15, SF.

7. Spotswood to Mallory, Nov. 1, 1864, *ORN*, ser. 2, 2:758–60; Medical journal, CSS *Atlanta*, Confederate States of America: Medical Records, McCain Library and Archives.

8. Spotswood to Mallory, Nov. 1, 1864, *ORN*, ser. 2, 2:758–60; Mitchell to S.S. Lee, Aug. 9, 1864, *ORN*, ser. 1, 10:730–31.

9. Register of Confederate Naval Patients in the C.S. Hospital Ship "St. Philip" at New Orleans, Louisiana, 1861–1862, and Register of Confederate Naval Patients in the Charity Hospital at New Orleans, Louisiana, 1861, Papers of Lewis Willis Minor, Albert and Shirley Small Special Collections Library; Medical journal, CSS *Gaines*, microfilm M1091, roll 15.

Notes—Chapter 11

10. Herrick, "Quinine as a Therapeutic Agent," 624–31.

11. Medical journal, CSS *Gaines*, roll 15, SF; Logan, "Prophylactic Effects of Quinine"; Merritt, "Quinine as a Prophylactic in Malarious Regions"; Herrick, "Quinine as a Therapeutic Agent," 618.

12. John Bell, "Report on the Materia Medica," 1089–92; Hasegawa, "Quinine Substitutes."

13. Voucher for Purcell, Ladd & Co., Aug. 29, 1863, and voucher for F.H. Robertson, Oct 1, 1863, roll 15, SF; Spotswood, enclosure, Nov. 30, 1863, *ORN*, ser. 1, 2:562; George B. Wood and Bache, *Dispensatory of the United States*, 347–48, 1297–98; Confederate States Army Medical Department, *Standard Supply Table of Indigenous Remedies*.

14. George B. Wood and Bache, *Dispensatory of the United States*, 112–13, 352–54; Voucher for Purcell, Ladd & Co., Dec. 20, 1861, roll 15, SF; Trent, "Apocynum Cannabinum"; Compiled service record for Trent, roll 250, microfilm M331, RG 109; Unit information, 2nd Regiment Virginia State Reserves, roll 383, microfilm M324, RG 109.

15. George B. Wood, *Treatise on Therapeutics and Pharmacology*, 316–17; George B. Wood and Bache, *Dispensatory of the United States*, 956–57; Gibbes diary, July 21, 1862.

16. "Antidote for Intermittent Fever," *Daily Constitutionalist* (Augusta, GA), July 25, 1861, 1; Phillips, "Indian Corn in Intermittent Fever"; "Corn as an Antiperiodic'; Ramsay, "Indigenous Remedies of the South"; Hasegawa, "Quinine Substitutes."

17. Medical journal, CSS *Gaines*, roll 15, SF.

18. Medical journals, CSS *General Polk* and CSS *Atlanta*, Confederate States of America: Medical Records, McCain Library and Archives; Hasegawa, "We Got Up and Began to Pack Our Medicines," 294.

19. Dunglison, *Medical Lexicon*, 800–801; CSND, *Instructions for the Guidance*, 24–26; Bollet, "Rheumatic Diseases among Civil War Troops."

20. Medical journal, CSS *Gaines*, roll 15 SF, Medical journals, CSS *Polk* and CSS *Atlanta*, Confederate States of America: Medical Records, McCain Library and Archives; George B. Wood and Bache, *Dispensatory of the United States*, 1222; George B. Wood, *Treatise on Therapeutics*, 337, 349–50.

21. Medical journals, CSS *General Polk* and CSS *Atlanta*, Confederate States of America: Medical Records, McCain Library and Archives; Medical journal, CSS *Gaines*, roll 15, SF; Confederate States Army Medical Department, *Standard Supply Table of the Indigenous Remedies*; Voucher for Purcell, Ladd & Co., Nov. 1, 1862, roll 15, SF; George B. Wood and Bache, *Dispensatory of the United States*, 473–75.

22. Bollet, *Civil War Medicine*, 296–304; Commentary, *Wilmington (NC) Journal*, Nov. 27 1862, 4; Charles J. Helm to Judah P. Benjamin, Sept. 3, 1862, *ORN*, ser. 1, 1:760–61; Extracts from Maffitt journal, Aug. 7–Sept. 1, 1862, *ORN*, ser. 1, 1:764–66; Wise, *Lifeline of the Confederacy*, 191–92.

23. Gibbes diary, Aug. 29 and Nov. 20, 1864; Ewart obituary, *Charleston Daily Courier*, October 14, 1864, 2.

24. Gibbes diary, Aug. 20–28, 1862.

25. James F. Harrison to surgeon in charge, General Hospital No. 21, and James E. Lindsay to unknown, Dec. 9, 1862, roll 15, SF; Carrington, statistics of the variolous diseases, Jan. 16, 1863, vol. 416, ch. 6, RG 109.

26. Hicks, "Scabrous Matters"; USND, *Instructions for the Government* (1857), 15.

27. Hicks, "Scabrous Matters."

28. Medical journals, CSS *General Polk* and CSS *Atlanta*, Confederate States of America: Medical Records, McCain Library and Archives; Medical journal, CSS *Gaines*, roll 15, SF; Register of Patients in the C.S. Hospital Ship *St. Philip* at New Orleans, Louisiana, and Register of Naval Patients in the Charity Hospital at New Orleans, Papers of Lewis Willis Minor, Albert and Shirley Small Special Collections Library; George B. Wood and Bache, *Dispensatory of the United States*, 1093. "Journal of Charles E. Lining, C.S.S. Shenandoah."

Notes—Chapter 12

29. Medical journal, CSS *Gaines*, Jan. 3–14, 1863, roll 15, SF.; James R. Dowell to John H. Reagan, October 16 and 25, 1861, with endorsements, roll 13, microfilm M437, RG 109; Joseph LeConte to Aaron Snowden Piggot, Sept. 28, 1863, Papers of Aaron Snowden Piggot, RG 109, NARA.

30. Medical journal, CSS *Gaines*, June 16, 1863, roll 15 SF; Medical journal, CSS *Atlanta*, Mar. 29–Apr. 11, 1862, Confederate States of America: Medical Records, McCain Library and Archives.

31. Rations, Provisional Navy of the Confederate States, roll 51, SF; Semmes, *Memoirs of Service Afloat*, 159, 230; Medical journal, CSS *Gaines*, roll 15, SF; Stevens and Leader, "Skeletal Remains."

32. Gibbes diary, Apr. 7–10, 1861.

33. Gibbes diary, Apr. 7–10, 1861; G.R.B. Horner, *Diseases and Injuries of Seamen*, 151–52; Wilson, *Naval Hygiene*, 34–38.

34. G.R.B. Horner, *Diseases and Injuries of Seamen*, 151–52, 244; Wilson, *Naval Hygiene*, 34–38.

35. Stevens and Leader, "Skeletal Remains"; "Journal of Charles E. Lining, C.S.S. Shenandoah."

36. "Journal of Charles E. Lining, C.S.S. Shenandoah"; Whitecar, *Four Years aboard the Whaleship*, 99.

37. Sinclair, Harrison, and Carrington to Spotswood, Aug. 26, 1864, *ORN*, ser. 1, 10:735–36; Spotswood to Mallory, Nov. 1, 1864, *ORN*, ser. 2, 2:758–60; Wilkes to Gideon Welles, Aug. 15, 1862; *ORN*, ser. 1, 7:651–52; Letterman, *Medical Recollections of the Army of the Potomac*, 13–14; Chisolm, *Manual of Military Surgery*, 32–33.

38. "Journal of Charles E. Lining, C.S.S. Shenandoah."

Chapter 12

1. USND, *Instructions for the Government* (1857), 9–10.

2. CSND, *Register ... to January 1*, 1863; CSND, *Register ... to January 1, 1864*; CSND, *Regulations*, 163; Notice, *Charleston Mercury*, Oct. 2, 1862, 2; William L. Bradford, notice, *Daily Picayune* (New Orleans), May 28, 1861, 3; C. Manigault Morris, notice, *Daily News* (Savannah), Feb. 13, 1862, 2; French Forrest, notice, *Daily Richmond Whig*, May 5, 1862, 3.

3. Gibbes journal, Feb. 21, 1861.

4. CSND, *Regulations*, 125, 170–71.

5. CSND, *Register ... to January 1, 1864*; Thomas R. Ware, pay list, June 30, 1864, roll 17, SF; Muster and pay rolls, CSS *United States*, roll 19, MF; Muster and pay rolls, CSS *Sampson*, roll 18, MF; Gibbes diary, Nov. 1, 1862; "Letter from 'The Ancient Mariner,'" *New Orleans Weekly Crescent*, June 1, 1861, 6; James D. Johnston to G. Floyd Johnston, Oct. 19, 1861, roll 19, SF. Darby also served on the commerce raider *Sumter* ("The Escape of the Pirate Sumter from the Iroquois," *Boston Morning Journal*, Jan. 13, 1862, 2).

6. Act of April 16, 1862, ch. 31, § 5, Cong. C.S.A. Stat. 29, 31 (1862); Thomas W. Brent to Charlton, July 9, 1862, ZB file for Charlton, Navy Department Library.

7. Act of May 1, 1863, ch. 68, Cong. C.S.A. Stat. 153 (1863); Josiah Tatnall to Stoakley, June 24, 1863, and Lee to Mallory, Oct. 31, 1864, *ORN*, ser. 2, 2:753–55.

8. Cooper to Joseph E. Johnston, Mar. 22, 1864, John K. Mitchell to W.W. Hunter, Mar. 26, 1864, Hunter to Carnes, Apr. 1, 1864, and Carnes to Hunter, Apr. 13, 1864, *ORN*, ser. 1, 15:720–22, 725–26.

9. Gibbes diary, Aug. 15, 1864.

10. CSND, *Regulations*, 4–6; Wells, *Confederate Navy*, 18–27.

11. Minor, *Confederate Naval Cadet*, 141–63; Scharf, *History of the Confederate States Navy*, 774; Officers of the Board, and Mallory to G.N. Hollins, June 19 and 24, 1862, vol. 294, ch. 8, RG 109; Voucher for Harrison, Apr. 13, 1863, roll 19, SF; Morgan, "Realistic War College."

12. CSND, *Instructions for Guidance*, 6; CSND, *Regulations*, 16; Charleton to Jones, Dec. 19, 1862, Tattnall to Freeman, Ford, and Emory, Dec. 20, 1862, and Freeman, Ford, and Emory to Tattnall, Dec. 20, 1862, roll 16, SF; G.R.B. Horner, *Diseases and Injuries of Seamen*, 14.

13. Act of Feb. 17, 1864, ch. 56, C.S.A. Stat. 203 (1864); Act of June 7, 1864, ch. 21, C.S.A. Stat. 230 (1864).

Notes—Chapter 13

14. John R.F. Tattnall to S.A. Durham, Jan. 27, 1865, with endorsements, and certificate of disability for retiring of invalid soldiers, Jan. 31, 1865, roll 16, SF.

15. John K. Mitchell to McClenahan, Aug. 24, 1863, ZB file for McClenahan, Navy Department Library; Hasegawa, "Officers' Promotions."

16. CSND, *Regulations*, 175; S.W. Averett et al., to John N. Maffitt, Jan. 23, 1863, *ORN*, ser. 1, 2:640; Maffitt, journal extract for Jan. 23, 1863, *ORN*, ser. 1, 2:668; Maffitt, log extract for Jan. 23, 1863, *ORN*, ser. 1, 2:674.

17. Mitchell, inspection order, Jan. 16, 1865, roll 17, SF; CSND, *Regulations*, 51, 52.

18. Harrison et al. to Mitchell, June 17, 1864, ORN, ser. 1, 10:702; Morgan, "Realistic War College"; Scharf, *History of the Confederate States Navy*, 775; CSND, *Regulations*, 178.

19. Sinclair et al. to Spotswood, Aug. 26, 1864, *ORN*, ser. 1, 10:735–36.

20. George N. Hollins to Greenhow, June 6, 1861, *ORN*, ser. 1, 10:24–25.

21. Article 43, Code of Regulations, in *Report of the Secretary of the Navy*, Dec. 6, 1858, H.R. Exec. Doc. 2, 35th Cong., 2nd sess., 226 (1858); CSND, general order, Jan. 13, 1863, *Richmond Enquirer*, Jan. 16, 1863, 2; Amicus [pseud.], "A Card," *Richmond Whig and Public Advertiser*, Jan. 20, 1863, 2; Hasegawa, "Consequential Incident."

22. *Ibid.*; "A Strange Proceeding," *Richmond Whig and Public Advertiser*, Jan. 20, 1863, 1; "Mr. Mallory—Strange Conduct," *Semi-Weekly Standard* (Raleigh, NC), Jan. 23, 1863, 4; Item, *Western Democrat* (Charlotte, NC), Jan. 27, 1863, 3; Hollins, extracts from notes and list of officers and men, *ORN*, ser. 1, 4:553–55; French Forrest to D.B. Conrad, Dec. 30, 1862, ZB file for Conrad, Navy Department Library; CSND, *Register ... to January 1, 1864*, 38.

23. Mallory to Van Benthuysen, Jan. 13, 1863, A.C. Van Benthuysen Papers, Louisiana Historical Association Collection.

24. "Confederate States Congress," *Daily Richmond Enquirer*, Jan. 21, 1863, 2; "Confederate Congress," *Richmond Whig and Public Advertiser*, Mar. 31, 1863, 2; "Confederate Congress," *Daily Richmond Examiner*, Apr. 29, 1863; Report on Senate bill S. 4, Apr. 28, 1863, *JCCSA*, 6:448.

25. John K. Mitchell to Pegram, June 19, 1863, and voucher for Sands, July 18, 1863, roll 21, and voucher for W.H. Belden, Sept. 30, 1863, roll 14, SF; Muster and pay rolls, CSS *Selma*, 4th qtr. 1863, roll 167, MF.

Chapter 13

1. Hollins, extracts from notes, *ORN*, ser. 1, 4:553–55.

2. CSND, *Ordnance Instructions*, 101, 106; Douglas, *Treatise on Naval Gunnery*, 514–15.

3. Conrad, "Capture and Burning of the Federal Gunboat 'Underwriter'"; Muster and pay rolls, Richmond, 1st qtr. 1864, roll 172, MF.

4. Joseph Price to Hunter, June 8, 1864, Hunter to S.S. Lee, June 9, 1864, and Pierson to John A. Dahlgren, Sept. 10, 1864, *ORN*, ser. 1, 15:481–88, 500, 501–2; Minor, *Confederate Naval Cadet*, 90–97.

5. Wood to S.R. Mallory, Sept. 7, 1863, *ORN*, ser. 1, 5:344–45.

6. Minor, *Confederate Naval Cadet*, 114–15; R.D. Minor to Franklin Buchanan, Feb. 2, 1864, *ORN*, ser. 1, 2:822–28.

7. Abstract log of CSS *Florida*, Jan. 16–May 1, 1863, *ORN*, ser. 1, 2:673–83.

8. Cushing, "Destruction of the 'Albemarle,'" D.H. Hill, *North Carolina*, 489–90; CSND, *Regulations*, 5.

9. Phillips, "Career of the Merrimac," 605–6.

10. Gibbes diary, Nov. 7, and Dec. 16 and 18, 1861.

11. Tatnall to Jeffery, June 28, 1864, ZB file for Jeffery, Navy Department Library.

12. Semmes, *Memoirs of Service Afloat*, 817–23.

13. Muster roll, Naval Brigade, roll 43, SF.

14. Rochelle, *Life of Rear Admiral John*

Notes—Chapter 14 and Conclusion

Randolph Tucker, 51–55; Eanes, *Captured at Sailor's Creek*, 77–78; "At the War's Close: Report of Sailors' Creek Battle, April 7th, 1865," *Morning Post* (Raleigh, NC), May 14, 1905, 9; "Paroles of the Army of Northern Virginia," 449–50; Sinclair, *Two Years on the Alabama*, 314–15; Hotchkiss, *Virginia*, 920–21; Evans, *Confederate Military History*, 546–47.

Chapter 14

1. "Richmond As It Is," *World* (New York), Apr. 7, 1865, 1; Calcutt, *Richmond's Wartime Hospitals*, 187; "Mr. Theodore C. Wilson's Dispatches," *New York Herald*, Apr. 13, 1865, 5.

2. Paroles, roll 44, SF; CSN Prisoners of War, roll 16, SF; Wheeden to Andrew Johnson, July 26, 1865, roll 30, microfilm M1003, RG 94; Hasegawa, *Matchless Organization*, 174–76.

3. Muster roll, Naval Brigade, roll 43, SF; Semmes, *Memoirs of Service Afloat*, 822–23, Paroles, roll 44, SF.

4. Spotswood to Andrew Johnson, June 28 and Aug 23, 1865, Spotswood to unknown, Feb. 24, 1867, and F.U. Still to Stanbery, May 14, 1867, microfilm roll 15, microfilm M1003, RG 94; Abraham Lincoln, proclamation, Dec. 8, 1863, 13 Stat. 737 (1866); Andrew Johnson, proclamation, May 29, 1865, 13 Stat. 758 (1866); Hasegawa, *Matchless Organization*, 138.

5. Gibbes diary, Apr. 14–June 9, 1865.

6. *National Cyclopaedia of American Biography*, 16–17; "Death of Dr. Charles E. Lining," *News and Courier* (Charleston), Mar. 2, 1897, 3.

7. Kelly and Burrage, *American Medical Biographies*, 519–20; Conrad, "Capture and Burning of the Federal Gunboat 'Underwriter,'" "Capture of the C.S. Ram Tennessee," and "History of the First Battle of Manassas"; Phillips, "Career of the Merrimac"; Booth to Superintendent of Naval War Records, Oct. 3, 1898, ZB file for Booth, Navy Department Library; USND, *Officers in the Confederate States Navy*, 15; Kell, *Recollections of a Naval Life*, 291–93; Haywood, "Life on the 'Alabama'"; "Life on the *Alabama*" [editor's note]; Garretson, "Sensation as a Mode of Motion"; Garretson, "Vibration of Rocks."

8. Hargis, "Sketch of the History of Quarantine"; "Convention of Ex-Confederate Surgeons"; "Personal and General Notes," *Daily Picayune* (New Orleans), Sept. 10, 1884, 2; "One of Washington's Swords," *Bloomington (IN) Telephone*, May 17, 1889, 2; "Death of Dr. William A.W. Spotswood," *Daily Register* (Mobile), Sept. 8, 1891, 4.

Conclusion

1. "The Grand Campaign," *World* (New York), Apr. 8, 1865, 1, 8; Beers, *Confederacy*, 338.

2. *Medical and Surgical History*; Spotswood to Mallory, Nov. 30, 1863, Apr. 28, 1864, and Nov. 1, 1864, *ORN*, ser. 2, 2:559–61, 647, 758–60.

3. Spotswood to Mallory, Nov. 1, 1864, *ORN*, ser. 2, 2:758–60.

4. Hasegawa, *Matchless Organization*, 84–94, 107–25; Rochard, "Surgical Service," May 17, 1862, 272.

5. Franklin Buchanan to Mallory, Aug. 13, 1864, file N355, roll 77, microfilm M474, RG 109; John K. Mitchell to George E. Pickett, August 10, 1864, *ORN*, ser. 1, 10:731.

Bibliography

Archives

Albert and Shirley Small Special Collections Library, University of Virginia, Charlottesville, VA
- Papers of Lewis Willis Minor, MSS 3988

Georgia State Archives, Morrow, GA
- Incoming Correspondence, Adjutant General, 1861–1914

Library of Congress, Washington, D.C.
- Luther Guiteau Billings Articles and Photographs, 1865–1900
- Daniel B. Conrad Diaries, 1855–64

Louisiana Historical Association Collection, Howard–Tilton Memorial Library, Tulane University, New Orleans, LA
- A.C. Van Benthuysen Papers

McCain Library and Archives, Special Collections, University of Southern Mississippi, Hattiesburg, MS
- Confederate States of America: Medical Records

National Archives and Records Administration, Washington, D.C.
- Record Group 15: Records of the Veterans Administration
  - Microfiche M1274: Case Files of Disapproved Pension Applications of Widows and Other Dependents of Civil War and Later Navy Veterans
- Record Group 24: Records of the Bureau of Naval Personnel
  - Microfilm M330: Abstracts of Service Records of Naval Officers ("Records of Officers"), 1798–1893
- Record Group 29: Records of the Bureau of the Census
  - Microfilm M653: Eighth Census of the United States, 1860
- Record Group 45: Naval Records Collection of the Office of Naval Records and Library
  - Entry 137: Registers of Applications for Appointment as Assistant Surgeon, Oct. 1834–Nov. 1875
  - Entry 652: Payrolls of Civilian Employees at Confederate Shore Establishments, May 1861–Dec. 1864
  - Microfilm M148: Letters Received by the Secretary of the Navy from Commissioned Officers below the Rank of Commander and from Warrant Officers ("Officers' Letters"), 1802–84
  - Microfilm M625: Area File of the Naval Records Collection
  - Microfilm M1091: Subject File of the Confederate States Navy, 1861–65
  - Microfilm T829: Miscellaneous Records of the Office of Naval Records and Library
- Record Group 52: Records of the Bureau of Medicine and Surgery
  - Entry 43: Statements of Service of Medical Officers, 1842–73
- Record Group 94: Records of the Adjutant General's Office, 1780s–1917

Bibliography

- Microfilm M619: Letters Received by the Office of the Adjutant General (Main Series), 1861–70
- Microfilm M1003: Case Files of Applications from Former Confederates for Presidential Pardons ("Amnesty Papers")
- Record Group 109: War Department Collection of Confederate Records
  - Ch. 1, Vol. 6: Special Orders, Adjutant and Inspector General's Office, March–October 1, 1861
  - Ch. 1, Vol. 8: Special Orders, Adjutant and Inspector General's Office, January–March 1862
  - Ch. 6, Vol. 416: Letters Sent, Medical Director's Office, Richmond, 1862–63
  - Ch. 6, Vol. 557: Reports of the Board for Examining Hospital Stewards, 1863–64
  - Ch. 6, Vol. 665: Register of Patients, Way and Yandell Hospitals and Meridian, 1865
  - Ch. 7, Vol. 19: Register of Bills Sent to the Senate by the House, May 1864–March 1865
  - Ch. 8, Vol. 294: Record of the Board for Examining Midshipmen, 1861–62
  - Entry 160: Miscellaneous Records Relating to the Navy, 1862–64
  - Entry 163: Congressional Bills and Resolutions
  - Entry 175: Memorials and Petitions, 1861–65
  - Microfilm M251: Compiled Service Records of Confederate Soldiers Who Served in Organizations from the State of Florida
  - Microfilm M260: Records Relating to Confederate Naval and Marine Personnel
  - Microfilm M266: Compiled Service Records of Confederate Soldiers Who Served in Organizations from the State of Georgia
  - Microfilm M269: Compiled Service Records of Confederate Soldiers Who Served in Organizations from the State of Mississippi
  - Microfilm M270: Compiled Service Records of Confederate Soldiers Who Served in Organizations from the State of North Carolina
  - Microfilm M311: Compiled Service Records of Confederate Soldiers Who Served in Organizations from the State of Alabama
  - Microfilm M324: Compiled Service Records of Confederate Soldiers Who Served in Organizations from the State of Virginia
  - Microfilm M331: Compiled Service Records of Confederate Generals and Staff Officers, and Nonregimental Enlisted Men
  - Microfilm M346: Confederate Papers Relating to Citizens or Business Firms
  - Microfilm M347: Unfiled Papers and Slips Belonging in Confederate Compiled Service Records
  - Microfilm M437: Letters Received by the Confederate Secretary of War, 1861–65
  - Microfilm M474: Letters Received by the Confederate Adjutant and Inspector General, 1861–1865
  - Papers of Aaron Snowden Piggot, M.D., 1874–99

National Civil War Naval Museum, Columbus, GA
- Diary of Dr. Robert Reeve Gibbes, 1861–65

National Library of Medicine, Bethesda, MD
- Examination Papers Collection, 1831–60, U.S Navy Department, Board of Medicine and Surgery.

Navy Department Library, Naval History and Heritage Command, Washington, D.C.
- ZB (Personnel) Files

Tompkins–McCaw Library, Special Collections and Archives, Virginia Commonwealth University, Richmond, VA
- Sanger Historical Files

Bibliography

U.S. Army Heritage and Education Center, Carlisle, PA
  • Civil War Photograph Collection, Military Order of the Loyal Legion of the United States, Massachusetts Commandery
Virginia Museum of History and Culture, Richmond, VA
  • Broadside Collection
Waring Historical Library, Medical University of South Carolina, Charleston, SC
  • Francis Peyre Porcher Papers

Articles and Books

"Association of Army and Navy Surgeons." *Confederate States Medical and Surgical Journal* 1, no. 1 (Jan. 1864): 13–16.

Becker, Joseph. "Fort Fisher and Wilmington." *Frank Leslie's Popular Monthly* 38, no. 2 (Aug. 1894): 230–39.

Beers, Henry Putney. *The Confederacy: A Guide to the Archives of the Government of the Confederate States of America.* Washington, D.C.: National Archives and Records Administration, 1986.

Bell, Andrew McIlwaine. *Mosquito Soldiers: Malaria, Yellow Fever, and the Course of the American Civil War.* Baton Rouge: Louisiana State University Press, 2010.

Bell, John. "Report on Materia Medica and Therapeutics for the Year 1857," pt. 2. *North American Medico-Chirurgical Review* 2, no. 6 (Nov. 1858): 1079–1103.

Blum, David A., and Nese F. DeBruyne. American War and Military Operations Casualties: Lists and Statistics. Congressional Research Service, RL 32492 (version 33), 2020.

Bollet, Alfred Jay. "Amputations in the Civil War." In *Years of Change and Suffering: Modern Perspectives on Civil War Medicine*, edited by James M. Schmidt and Guy R. Hasegawa, 57–67. Roseville, MN: Edinborough Press, 2009.

Bollet, Alfred Jay. *Civil War Medicine: Challenges and Triumphs.* Tucson: Galen Press, 2002.

Bollet, Alfred Jay. "Rheumatic Diseases among Civil War Troops." *Arthritis and Rheumatism* 34, no. 9 (September 1991): 1197–1203.

Brewer, William A., Samuel M. Colcord, Evan T. Ellis, and John I. Thomsen. "Report of the Committee on the Drug Market." *Proceedings of the American Pharmaceutical Association at the Fifteenth Annual Meeting, Held at New Work City, September, 1867,* 267–307. Philadelphia: Merrihew and Sons, 1867.

Butcher, Bernard L., ed. *Genealogical and Personal History of the Upper Monongahela Valley, West Virginia,* Vol. 3. New York: Lewis Historical Publishing, 1912.

Butters' Richmond Directory for 1855. Richmond: H.K. Ellyson's Steam Presses, 1855.

Calcutt, Rebecca Barbour. *Richmond's Wartime Hospitals.* Gretna, LA: Pelican, 2005.

Callahan, Edward W., ed. *List of Officers of the Navy of the United States and of the Marine Corps from 1775 to 1900.* New York: L.R. Hamersly, 1901.

Campbell, R. Thomas. *Confederate Ironclads at War.* Jefferson, NC: McFarland, 2019.

Canney, Donald L. *Lincoln's Navy: The Ships, Men and Organization, 1861–65.* Annapolis: Naval Institute Press, 1998.

Carney, Charles T., A.P. Sharp, Edward R. Squibb, and A.B. Taylor. "Report on Home Adulterations." In *Proceedings of the American Pharmaceutical Association at the Eighth Annual Meeting, Held in Boston, Mass. September, 1859,* 245–64. Boston: Geo. C. Rand and Avery, 1859.

Chenowith M., and C.J. Mock. "Hurricane 'Amanda': Rediscovery of a Forgotten

Bibliography

U.S. Civil war Florida Hurricane." *Bulletin of the American Meteorological Society* 94, no. 11 (Nov. 2013): 1735–42.

Chisolm, J. Julian. *A Manual of Military Surgery.* 3rd ed. Columbia, SC: Evans and Cogswell, 1864.

Chitwood, W.R. "Doctor Spotswood and the Confederate Navy." *Virginia Medical Monthly* 103, no. 10 (October 1976): 729–33.

Cole, W.H. "Manufacture and Consumption of Quinine in the United States." *Pharmaceutical Journal* 14 (July 1, 1854): 15–16.

"Commercial Dependence of the South on the North." *De Bow's Southern and Western Review* 12 (Mar. 1852): 299–300.

Confederate States Army Medical Department. *General Directions for Collecting and Drying Medicinal Substances of the Vegetable Kingdom.* Richmond: Surgeon General's Office, 1862.

Confederate States Army Medical Department. *Standard Supply Table of the Indigenous Remedies for Field Service, and the Sick in General Hospitals.* Richmond: Surgeon General's Office, 1863.

Confederate States Navy Department. *Confederate States Navy Register for 1862.* Richmond: Enquirer Book and Job Press, 1862.

Confederate States Navy Department. *Instructions for the Guidance of the Medical Officers of the Navy of the Confederate States.* Richmond: Macfarlane and Fergusson, 1864.

Confederate States Navy Department. *Ordnance Instructions for the Confederate States Navy Relating to the Preparation of Vessels of War for Battle.* 3rd ed. London: Saunders, Otley, and Co., 1864.

Confederate States Navy Department. *Register of the Commissioned and Warrant Officers of the Navy of the Confederate States to January 1, 1863.* Richmond: Macfarlane and Fergusson, 1862.

Confederate States Navy Department. *Register of the Commissioned and Warrant Officers of the Navy of the Confederate States to January 1, 1864.* Richmond: Macfarlane and Fergusson, 1864.

Confederate States Navy Department. *Register of the Officers of the Confederate Navy, 1862.* Richmond: Navy Department, 1862.

Confederate States Navy Department. *Regulations for the Navy of the Confederate States, 1862.* Richmond: Macfarlane and Fergusson, 1862.

Confederated Southern Memorial Association. *History of the Confederated Memorial Associations of the South.* New Orleans: Graham Press, 1904.

Conrad, Daniel B. "Capture and Burning of the Federal Gunboat 'Underwriter,' In the Neuse, off Newbern, N.C., in February, 1864." *Southern Historical Society Papers* 19 (Jan. 1891): 93–100.

Conrad, Daniel B. "Capture of the C.S. Ram Tennessee in Mobile Bay, August, 1864." *Southern Historical Society Papers* 19 (Jan. 1891): 72–82.

Conrad, Daniel B. "History of the First Battle of Manassas and the Organization of the Stonewall Brigade." *Southern Historical Society* Papers 19 (Jan. 1891): 82–92.

"Convention of Ex-Confederate Surgeons." *Atlanta Medical and Surgical Journal* 12, no. 3 (June 1874): 182–88.

"Corn as an Antiperiodic." *North American Medico-Chirurgical Review* 2, no. 5 (Sept. 1858): 970–71.

Coski, John M. *Capital Navy: The Men, Ships and Operations of the James River Squadron.* New York: Savas Beatie, 2005.

Cushing, W.B. "The Destruction of the 'Albemarle.'" In *Battles and Leaders of the Civil War,* edited by Robert Underwood Johnson and Clarence Clough Buel, Vol. 4, 634–41. New York: Century, 1884.

Davis, Jefferson. [Message to the President of the Congress, transmitting communications from all the departments, except the War Department], Feb. 15, 1862. Richmond, 1862.

Day, James M. "Leon Smith: Confederate Mariner." *East Texas Historical Journal* 3, no. 1 (Mar. 1965): 34–49.

Bibliography

"Deaths." *University of Maryland Bulletin of the School of Medicine* 9. no. 4 (April 1925): 169–70.

De Leon, Thomas Cooper. *Belles Beaux and Brains of the 60s*. New York: G.W. Dillingham, 1909.

Douglas, Howard. *A Treatise on Naval Gunnery*, 5th ed. London: John Murray, 1860.

Dudley, William S. *Going South: U.S. Navy Officer Resignations & Dismissals on the Eve of the Civil War*. Washington, D.C.: Naval Historical Foundation, 1981.

Dufour, Charles L. *The Night the War Was Lost*. Garden City, NY: Doubleday, 1960.

Dunglison, Robley. *Medical Lexicon: A Dictionary of Medical Science*. Philadelphia: Blanchard and Lee, 1860.

Eanes, Greg. *Captured at Sailor's Creek*. Vol. 1. N.p.: Eanes Group, 2015.

England, Joseph W. "The American Manufacture of Quinine Sulphate." *Alumni Report* (Philadelphia College of Pharmacy) 34 (Mar. 1898): 57–64.

Evans, Clement A., ed. *Confederate Military History: A Library of Confederate States History*, Extended Edition, Vol. 3. Wilmington, NC: Broadfoot, 1987–88.

"The First Alumnus of the University to Enter the Medical Corps of the Navy." *University of Virginia Bulletins*, n.s., 4, no. 2 (Apr. 1904): 54–55.

Freedley, Edwin T. *Philadelphia and Its Manufactures: A Hand-Book Exhibiting the Development, Variety, and Statistics of the Manufacturing Industry of Philadelphia in 1857*. Philadelphia: Edward Young, 1859.

Freedley, Edwin T., ed. *Leading Pursuits and Leading Men: A Treatise on the Principal Trades and Manufactures of the United States*. Philadelphia: Edward Young, 1854.

Freeman, Douglas Southall. *A Calendar of Confederate Papers*. Richmond: Confederate Museum, 1908.

Garretson, Frederic. "Sensation as a Mode of Motion." *Baltimore Medical Journal* 1, no. 8 (Aug. 1870): 449–56.

Garretson, Frederic. "Vibration of Rocks in Patapsco Valley, Maryland." *Popular Science Monthly* 20 (Feb. 1882): 541–43.

Gradijan, Leanne. "Navy Surgeons in the Civil War: A Statistical Report." *Grog* 5, no. 3 (Summer 2011): 28–29.

Hamilton, Frank Hastings. *A Practical Treatise on Military Surgery*. New York: Baillière Brothers, 1861.

Hargis, R.B.S. "Sketch of the History of Quarantine at Pensacola, Fla." *National Board of Health Bulletin* 3, no. 9 (Aug. 27, 1881): 63–64; no. 13 (Sept. 24, 1881): 95; no. 15 (Oct. 8, 1881): 111–12; no. 16 (Oct. 15, 1881): 119–20.

Hasegawa, Guy R. "A Consequential Incident at Drewry's Bluff." *Civil War Navy—The Magazine* 10, no. 3 (Winter 2023): 59–63.

Hasegawa, Guy R. *Matchless Organization: The Confederate Army Medical Department*. Carbondale: Southern Illinois University Press, 2021.

Hasegawa, Guy R. "Officers' Promotions in the Confederate Navy." *Civil War Navy—The Magazine* 11, no. 1 (Summer 2023): 21–37.

Hasegawa, Guy R. "Piscine Perils in Mobile Bay." *Civil War Navy—The Magazine* 11, no. 2 (Fall 2023): 56–62.

Hasegawa, Guy R. "Quinine Substitutes in the Confederate Army." *Military Medicine* 172, no. 6 (June 2007): 650–655.

Hasegawa, Guy R. "'We Got Up and Began to Pack Our Medicines': What Dr. Fulton Prescribed." In *Civil War Medicine: A Surgeon's Diary*, edited by Robert D. Hicks, 288–301. Bloomington: Indiana University Press, 2019.

Hasegawa, Guy R., and F. Terry Hambrecht. "The Confederate Medical Laboratories." *Southern Medical Journal* 96, no. 12 (Dec. 2003): 1221–30.

Haywood, P.D. "Life on the 'Alabama.'" *Century Magazine* 31, no. 6 (Apr. 1886): 901–10.

Herndon, G. Melvin. "The Confederate States Naval Academy." *Virginia Magazine of History and Biography* 69, no. 3 (July 1961): 300–323.

Herrick, S.S. "Quinine as a Therapeutic Agent." *Transactions of the American*

Bibliography

Medical Association 20 (1869): 583–636.

Hicks, Robert D. "Scabrous Matters: Spurious Vaccinations in the Confederacy." In *War Matters: Material Culture in the Civil War Era*, edited by Joan E. Cashin, 123–50. Chapel Hill: University of North Carolina Press. 2018.

Hill, D.H., Jr. *North Carolina*. Vol. 4 of *Confederate Military History*. Atlanta: Confederate Publishing, 1899.

Hill, Jim Dan. *The Civil War Sketchbook of Charles Ellery Stedman, Surgeon, United States Navy*. San Rafael, CA: Presidio Press, 1976.

Holden, J. "The Hospital Corps of the United States Navy." *Hospital Corps Quarterly* 10, no. 3 (July 1926): 1–16.

Homans, Benjamin. *Register of the Commissioned and Warrant Officers of the Navy of the United States, Including Officers of the Marine Corps. Corrected from Authentic Sources, to the 15th September, 1842*. Washington, D.C.: Alexander and Barnard, 1842.

Horner, Frederick. "The Medical Corps of the U.S. Navy." *Journal of the American Medical Association* 24, no. 10 (March 9, 1895): 347–49.

Horner, G.R.B. *Diseases and Injuries of Seamen: With Remarks on Their Enlistment, Naval Hygiene, and the Duties of Medical Officers*. Philadelphia: Lippincott, Grambo, 1854.

Hotchkiss, Jedediah. *Virginia*. Vol. 3 of *Confederate Military History*. Atlanta: Confederate Publishing, 1899.

Jeffery, Richard W. "Gun-shot Wound of Lung, Liver and Intestines." *Confederate States Medical and Surgical Journal* 1, no. 3 (March 1864): 39–40.

Jones, John B. *A Rebel War Clerk's Diary*. Edited by James I. Robertson, Jr. 2 vols. Lawrence: University Press of Kansas, 2015.

"Journal of Charles E. Lining, C.S.S. Shenandoah." In *A Calendar of Confederate Papers with a Bibliography of Some Confederate Publications*, edited by Douglas Southall Freeman, 126–63. Richmond: Confederate Museum, 1908.

Journal of the Congress of the Confederate States of America, 1861–1865. 7 vols. S. Doc. 234, 58th Cong., 2nd sess., 1904–5.

Kell, John McIntosh. "Cruise and Combats of the 'Alabama.'" *Century Magazine* 31, no. 6 (Apr. 1886): 911–22.

Kell, John McIntosh. *Recollections of a Naval Life, Including the Cruises of the Confederate States Steamers "Sumter" and "Alabama."* Washington, D.C.: Neale, 1900.

Kelly, Howard A., and Walter L. Burrage. *American Medical Biographies*. Baltimore: Norman, Remington, 1920.

Kenney, Edward C. "From the Log of the Red Rover 1862–1865: A History of the First U.S. Navy Hospital Ship." *Missouri Historical Review* 60, no. 1 (Oct. 1965): 31–49.

Koste, Jodi L. "'Medical School for a Nation': The Medical College of Virginia, 1860–1865." In *Years of Change and Suffering: Modern Perspectives on Civil War Medicine*, edited by James M. Schmidt and Guy R. Hasegawa, 13–35. Roseville, MN: Edinborough Press, 2009.

Lamb, William. "The Defense of Fort Fisher." In *Battles and Leaders of the Civil War*, edited by Robert Underwood Johnson and Clarence Clough Buel, Vol. 4, 642–54. New York: Century, 1884.

Langley, Harold D. *A History of Medicine in the Early U.S. Navy*. Baltimore: Johns Hopkins University Press, 1995.

Lee, F.D., and J.L. Agnew. *Historical Record of the City of Savannah*. Savannah: J.H. Estill, 1869.

Letterman, Jonathan. *Medical Recollections of the Army of the Potomac*. New York: D. Appleton, 1866.

"Life on the *Alabama*" [editor's note]. *Century Magazine* 33, no. 5 (Mar. 1887): 805.

Logan, Samuel. "Prophylactic Effects of Quinine." *Confederate States Medical and Surgical Journal* 1, no. 6 (June 1864): 81–83.

Luraghi, Raimondo. *A History of the Confederate Navy*. Translated by Paolo E. Coletta. Annapolis: Naval Institute Press, 1996.

Bibliography

Lynch, John S. "Civil War Federal Navy Physicians." *Military Medicine* 168, no. 12 (Dec. 2003): 1044–48.

Lynch, John S. "Confederate Navy Medicine." *Military Medicine* 164, no. 11 (Nov. 1999): 809–13.

Lynn, John Worth. *Confederate Commando and Fleet Surgeon: Dr. Daniel B. Conrad.* Shippensburg, PA: Burd Street, 2001.

McLain, Minor H. "The Military Prison at Fort Warren." *Civil War History* 8, no. 2 (June 1962): 136–51.

The Medical and Surgical History of the War of the Rebellion. 3 vols. Washington, D.C.: Government Printing Office, 1870–88.

"Medical Service, United States Navy." *Boston Medical and Surgical Journal* 62, no. 20 (June 14, 1860): 415–16.

Melton, Maurice. *The Best Station of Them All: The Savannah Squadron, 1861–1865.* Tuscaloosa: University of Alabama Press, 2012.

Merritt, J. King. "Quinine as a Prophylactic in Malarious Regions." *American Medical Times* 3, no. 19 (Nov. 9, 1861): 305–6.

Minor, Hubbard T. *Confederate Naval Cadet: The Diary and Letters of Midshipman Hubbard T. Minor, with a History of the Confederate Naval Academy.* Edited by T. Thomas Campbell. Jefferson, NC: McFarland, 2007.

Moore, Frank. *The Rebellion Record: A Diary of American Events*, Vol. 9. New York: D. Van Nostrand, 1866.

Morgan, James Morris. "A Realistic War College." *United States Naval Institute Proceedings* 42, no. 162 (Mar.–Apr. 1916): 543–54.

National Cyclopaedia of American Biography. Vol. 19. New York: James T. White, 1926.

A Naval Encyclopedia. Philadelphia: L.R. Hamersly, 1884.

Nichols, F.B. "Review of the New York Markets, from March 24th to April 24th, 1861." *American Druggists' Circular and Chemical Gazette* 5 (May 1861): 112.

O'Brien, Thomas M., and Oliver Diefendorf. *General Orders of the War Department, Embracing the Years 1861, 1862 & 1863.* Vol. 1. New York: Derby and Miller, 1864.

Official Records of the Union and Confederate Navies in the War of the Rebellion. 30 vols. in 2 ser. Washington, D.C.: Government Printing Office, 1894–1922.

Ordinances Adopted by the Convention of Virginia in Secret Session, in April and May, 1861. Richmond: Wyatt M. Elliott, 1861.

Parker, William Harwar. "The Confederate States Navy." In *Confederate Military History*, Vol. 12, 1–115. Atlanta: Confederate Publishing, 1899.

Parker, William Harwar. *Recollections of a Naval Officer, 1841–1865.* New York: Charles Scribners' Sons, 1883.

"Paroles of the Army of Northern Virginia." *Southern Historical Society Papers* 15 (1887): 1–487.

Paullin, Charles Oscar. "Naval Administration." *Proceedings of the United States Naval Institute* 33, no. 4 (Dec. 1907): 1435–77.

Phillips, Dinwiddie B. "The Career of the Merrimac." *Southern Bivouac* 2, no. 10 (Mar. 1887): 598–605.

Phillips, Dinwiddie B. "Indian Corn in Intermittent Fever." *American Journal of the Medical Sciences*, n.s., 34, no. 68 (Oct. 1857): 554–55.

Porcher, Francis Peyre. *Resources of the Southern Fields and Forests.* Charleston, SC: Evans and Cogswell, 1863.

Porter, David D. *The Naval History of the Civil War.* New York: Sherman, 1886.

Ramsay, H.A. "Indigenous Remedies of the South for Intermittent Fever." *Nelson's Northern Lancet and American Journal of Medical Jurisprudence* 6, no. 3 (Dec. 1852): 147–48.

Read, Charles W. "Reminiscences of the Confederate States Navy." *Southern Historical Society Papers* 1, no. 5 (May 1876): 331–62.

Roberts, John C. "What Is a 'Naval Station'?" *JAG Journal*, Apr. 1951, 14–17.

Robertson, James I., ed. *Proceedings of the Advisory Council of the State of Virginia.* Richmond: Virginia State Library, 1977.

Bibliography

Rochard, Jules. "Surgical Service of the Navy in Times of War," *American Medical Times* 4 (May 17, 1862): 272–73; (May 24, 1862): 288–89; (May 31, 1862): 300–301.

Rochelle, James Henry. *Life of Rear Admiral John Randolph Tucker*. Washington, D.C.: Neale, 1903.

[Ruschenberger, William S.W.]. *A Brief History of an Existing Controversy on the Subject of Assimilated Rank in the Navy of the United States*. Philadelphia: G. Sherman, 1850.

[Ruschenberger, William S.W.]. Review of *Outlines of Naval Surgery*, by John Wilson. *American Journal of the Medical Sciences*, n.s. 12, no. 14 (Oct. 1846): 407–25.

Scharf, J. Thomas. *History of the Confederate States Navy*. New York: Rogers and Sherwood, 1887.

Semmes, Raphael. *Memoirs of Service Afloat, during the War between the States*. Baltimore: Kelly, Piet and Co., 1869.

Sheehy, Barry, and Cindy Wallace. *Savannah: Immortal City*. Vol. 1, *Civil War Savannah*. Austin, TX: Emerald Book Co., 2011.

Silverstone, Paul H. *Civil War Navies, 1855–1883*. Annapolis: Naval Institute Press, 2001.

Sinclair, Arthur. *Two Years on the Alabama*. 3rd ed. Boston: Lee and Shepard, 1896.

Sternberg, George M. "Fort Barrancas, Florida." In *A Report on the Hygiene of the United States Army* (Circular no. 8, Surgeon General's Office, War Department). Washington, D.C.: Government Printing Office, 1875.

Stevens, William D., and Jonathan M. Leader. "Skeletal Remains from the Confederate Naval Sailor and Marines' Cemetery, Charleston, SC." *Historical Archaeology* 40, no. 3 (2006): 74–88.

Still, William N., Jr., ed. *The Confederate Navy: The Ships, Men and Organization, 1861–65*. London: Conway Maritime Press, 1997.

The Stranger's Guide and Official Directory for the City of Richmond. Richmond: Geo. P. Evans, 1863.

Sullivan, David M. *Marines of the Civil War: The Officers, Honors, Records, and Regulations*. Morrisville, NC: Lulu, 2019.

"The Surgeon of the Alabama." *Lancet* 1 (June 25, 1864): 730.

Tomblin, Barbara Brooks. *Life in Jefferson Davis' Navy*. Annapolis: Naval Institute Press, 2019.

Trent, Peterfield. "Apocynum Cannabinum, as an Antiperiodic in the Treatment of Intermittents." *Southern Medical and Surgical Journal* n.s. 15, no. 1 (Jan. 1859): 6–10.

United States Navy Department. *Dictionary of American Naval Fighting Ships*, Vol. 2. Washington, D.C.: Government Printing Office, 1969.

United States Navy Department. *Instructions for the Government of the Medical Officers of the Navy of the United States*. Washington, D.C.: Alexander and Barnard, 1844.

United States Navy Department. *Instructions for the Government of the Medical Officers of the Navy of the United States*. Washington, D.C.: A.O.P. Nicholson, 1857.

United States Navy Department. *Officers in the Confederate States Navy, 1861–65*. Washington, D.C.: Government Printing Office, 1898.

United States Navy Department. *Register of Officers of the Confederate States Navy, 1861–1865*. Washington, D.C.: Government Printing Office, 1931.

United States Navy Department. *Register of the Commissioned and Warrant Officers of the Navy of the United States, Including Officers of the Marine Corps, and Others, for the Year 1845*. Washington, D.C.: C. Alexander, 1845.

United States Navy Department. *Register of the Commissioned and Warrant Officers of the Navy of the United States, Including Officers of the Marine Corps, and Others, for the Year 1853*. Washington, D.C.: C. Alexander, 1853.

United States Navy Department. *Register of the Commissioned and Warrant Officers of the Navy of the United States, Including Officers of the Marine Corps, and Others, for the Year 1854*.

Bibliography

Washington, D.C.: Robert Armstrong, 1854.

United States Navy Department. *Register of the Commissioned and Warrant Officers of the Navy of the United States, Including Officers of the Marine Corps, and Others, for the Year 1855.* Washington, D.C.: A.O.P. Nicholson, 1855.

United States Navy Department. *Register of the Commissioned and Warrant Officers of the Navy of the United States, Including Officers of the Marine Corps, and Others, for the Year 1856.* Washington, D.C.: A.O.P. Nicholson, 1856.

United States Navy Department. *Register of the Commissioned and Warrant Officers of the Navy of the United States, Including Officers of the Marine Corps, and Others, for the Year 1857.* Washington, D.C.: A.O.P. Nicholson, 1857.

United States Navy Department. *Register of the Commissioned and Warrant Officers of the Navy of the United States, Including Officers of the Marine Corps, and Others, for the Year 1858.* Washington, D.C.: William A. Harris, 1858.

United States Navy Department. *Register of the Commissioned and Warrant Officers of the Navy of the United States, Including Officers of the Marine Corps, and Others, for the Year 1859.* Washington, D.C.: William A. Harris, 1859.

United States Navy Department. *Register of the Commissioned and Warrant Officers of the Navy of the United States, Including Officers of the Marine Corps and Others, for the Year 1860.* Washington, D.C.: n.p., 1860.

United States Navy Department. *Register of the Commissioned and Warrant Officers of the Navy of the United States, Including Officers of the Marine Corps and Others, for the Year 1861.* Washington, D.C.: George W. Bowman, 1861.

United States Navy Department. *Register of the Commissioned, Warrant, and Volunteer Officers of the Navy of the United States, Including Officers of the Marine Corps and Others, to January 1, 1863.* Washington, D.C.: Government Printing Office, 1863.

United States Navy Department. *Register of the Commissioned, Warrant, and Volunteer Officers of the Navy of the United States, Including Officers of the Marine Corps and Others, to January 1, 1864.* Washington, D.C.: Government Printing Office, 1864.

United States Navy Department. *Register of the Commissioned, Warrant, and Volunteer Officers of the Navy of the United States, Including Officers of the Marine Corps and Others, to January 1, 1865.* Washington, D.C.: Government Printing Office, 1865.

United States Navy Department. *Regulations for the Government of the United States Navy. 1865.* Washington: Government Printing Office, 1865.

United States Navy Department. *Report of the Secretary of the Navy, with an Appendix, Containing Reports from Officers, December 1862.* Washington, D.C.: Government Printing Office, 1863.

United States Navy Department. *Report of the Secretary of the Navy, with an Appendix, Containing Reports from Officers, December, 1863.* Washington, D.C.: Government Printing Office, 1863.

United States Navy Department. *Uniform and Dress of the Confederate States.* Office Memorandum No. 7. Washington, D.C.: Government Printing Office, 1898.

United States War Department. *Revised Regulations for the Army of the United States, 1861.* Philadelphia: J.G.L. Brown, 1861.

Vanfelson, Charles A. *The Little Red Book or Department Directory.* Richmond: Tyler, Wise and Allegre, 1861.

"The Volunteer Navy in the Civil War." *United States Naval Institute Proceedings* 45, no. 10 (October 1919): 1691–94.

Wales, Philip S. *Sanitary and Statistical Report of the Surgeon-General of the Navy for the Year 1880.* Washington, D.C.: Government Printing Office, 1882.

Bibliography

The War of the Rebellion: A Compilation of the Official Records of the Union and Confederate Armies. 70 vols. in 4 ser. Washington, D.C.: Government Printing Office, 1880–1901.

Warren, Edward. *A Doctor's Experiences in Three Continents.* Baltimore: Cushings and Bailey, 1885.

Waterman, George S. "Notable Events of the Civil War." *Confederate Veteran* 7, no. 10 (Oct. 1899): 449–52.

Weidenmier, Marc D. "Turning Points in the U.S. Civil War: Views from the Grayback Market." *Southern Economic Journal* 68, no. 4 (April 2002): 875–90.

Wells, Tom Henderson. *The Confederate Navy: A Study in Organization.* Tuscaloosa: University of Alabama Press, 1971.

Whitecar, William B. Jr. *Four Years aboard the Whaleship.* Philadelphia: J.B. Lippincott, 1860.

Wilson, Joseph. *Naval Hygiene.* Washington, D.C.: Government Printing Office, 1870.

Wise, Stephen R. *Lifeline of the Confederacy: Blockade Running During the Civil War.* Columbia: University of South Carolina Press, 1988.

Wood, C.A., and F.B. Nichols. "Annual Report on Drugs for the Year 1860." In *Third Annual Report of the Chamber of Commerce of the State of New York, for the Year 1860–'61,* 303–09. New York: John W. Amerman, 1861.

Wood, C.A., and F.B. Nichols. "Review of the Drug Trade of New York." In *Fourth Annual Report of the Chamber of Commerce of the State of New York, for the Year 1861–'62,* 164–72. New York: John W. Amerman, 1862.

Wood, George B. *A Treatise on Therapeutics, and Pharmacology or Materia Medica.* Vol. 2. Philadelphia: J.B. Lippincott, 1856.

Wood, George B., and Franklin Bache. *The Dispensatory of the United States of America,* 11th ed. Philadelphia: J.B. Lippincott, 1858.

Wood, John Taylor. "The First Fight of Iron-Clads." *Century Magazine* 29, no. 5 (Mar. 1885): 738–54.

Woodworth, John M. *First Annual Report of the Supervising Surgeon of the Marine Hospital Service of the United States.* Washington, D.C.: Government Printing Office, 1872.

Zeilin, J.H. "Drug Business in the Late Confederate States." In *Proceedings of the National Wholesale Druggists Association, in Conventional at Indianapolis, Oct. 22, 23, 24, 25, 1889,* 182–86. Minneapolis: Swinburne, 1890.

Index

Numbers in ***bold italics*** refer to pages with illustrations

Addison, William J. 89, 93, 162, 191
African Americans 71, 88, 129
A.H. Schultz (steamer) 85
CSS *Alabama* 74, 90, ***102***, 103, 105, 181
CSS *Albemarle* 174
alcohol 121–22, 155–57
Allen, J.H. 74, 87
Ancrum, John L. 74
Andrews, John A. 79
apothecaries *see* medical purveying; stewards, surgeons' and hospital
Appomattox Court House, VA 176
Archer, Carthon 71–72
CSS *Arctic* 160
CSS *Arkansas* 73, 98, 99
Arkansas Post, AR 87, 88
army, Confederate 25, 26, 31; assisted by naval surgeons 78–80; medical officers 47; medical purveyors 113, 117, 118; as source of sailors 160–61; as source or destination of Confederate naval surgeons 44–46; *see also* hospitals, army
Association of Army and Navy Surgeons of the Confederate States 21
CSS *Atlanta* 66, 77, 94, 97; capture 105, 106; sickbay 141, 143, 148–49, 164; treatment of injured 103, 104, 154
Atsinger, Emile 131
Augusta, GA 122, 175, 179

Baker, Laurence S. 174
Baldwin, Robert T., Jr. 47, 191
CSS *Baltic* 78, 119
Banks, Robert Bruce 73
Barnett, J.A. 31
Barton, William P. C. 14, 63–64
batteries 85–89; Battery Brooke, VA 86; Battery Buchanan, AL 88; Battery Buchanan, NC 87; Battery Semmes,

VA; 86, 97; Cockpit Point, VA 87; Drewry's Bluff, VA 42, 65, 77, ***86***, 130, 139; Fort Fisher, NC 87; Mobile Bay, AL 88; St. Charles, AR 89; Ship Island, MS 89
Battle of Hampton Roads, VA 102, 127
Battle of Mobile Bay, AL ***84***, 100, 101, 106, 125, 131
Battle of Sailor's Creek, VA 176
Battle of St. Charles, AR 89
CSS *Beaufort* 99
Beauregard, P.G.T. 133
Beck, Morris B. 30
Becker, Joseph 87, ***88***
bedbugs 155
Belvin, James W. 166, 176, 191
Benedict, Noah Bennet 67
Benton, MS 132
Bermuda 90, 111, 114
Billings, Luther Guiteau 135
Billups, Mr. (slave owner) 129
Bishop, William S. 125
Blacknall, George 30, 38, 47, 127, 189
Bledsoe, Albert T. 16
blockade 22, 109, 110, 111, 114, 119–20
CSS *Bombshell* 105
Bondurant, Walter E. 44, 47, 93, 191
Bonham, Milledge L. 122
Bonner, Samuel Lafayette 47, 191
Booth, Edwin G. ***84***, ***180***, 181, 191; at Drewry's Bluff 85, 113; at Mobile Naval Hospital 131–32; as prisoner 105, 106, 126
Bowles, Richard C. ***84***, 85, 105, 106, 107, 126, 179, 191
Boxley, James G. 86, 97, 162, 176, 191
Boyd, William 31
Bracey, John R. 35
Brest, France 90, 112
Bright, Henry 129

231

Index

Brooklyn, NY 110, 114
Brown, Pike 85, 166, 191
Brown, Wyatt M. 25, 31
Buchanan, Franklin 102; commanding at Mobile, AL 53–54, 97, 144; wounded 100, 106, 125, 127, 128, 174–75
Bulloch, Irvine S. *180*
Bureau of Medicine and Surgery (Confederate Navy) 13–14, 15–22, 81, 94, 183–84, 186–87
Bureau of Medicine and Surgery (U.S. Navy) 13–15, 110
Butler, Benjamin F. 86, 139

Caire, Edward 81, 191
Carnes, W.W. 161
Carrington, William A. (army surgeon) 151
Carrington, William F. (naval surgeon) 17, 24, 85, 155, 159, 166, 189; at Pensacola, FL 81, 124, 125; service with Confederate army 78, 79, 80
casualties 2–3, 98–104; *see also* illness
catarrh 149
Chapman, Robert T. *51*
Charleston, SC 59, 71, 72, 77, 90, 143, 150, 153, 174, 187; hospital 64, 98, 132–33, 139, 150, 161; medical purveying 111, 113, 114, 115; naval station 77, 81, 114, 176; receiving ship 160; rendezvous 119, 159; squadron 83, 98, 115, 176
Charlotte, NC 133, 137, 164, 182
Charlton, Thomas J., Jr. 25, 30, 39, 47, 90, 105, 106, 160, 163, 190
CSS *Chattahoochee* 72, 104, 113, 123
Chester (Chesterville), SC 133
CSS *Chicora* 77, 98
Chisolm, J.J. 155
Christian, Marcellus P. 79, 102, 129, 190
Christmas, Henry 47, 191
City Hospital, Savannah, GA 72, 133–34
civilian physicians 69–75
Claiborne, Gregory W. 191
Claiborne, James F. 167–68
Cockpit Point, VA 87
Coggin, William W. 45–46, 179, 193, 204*n*27
Columbus, GA 104, 113, 123
Colzey, E.F. 123
commerce raiders 89–90; *see also* specific vessels

Confederate States Medical and Surgical Journal 22
Confederate States Naval Academy 139, 162, 164; *see also* CSS *Patrick Henry*
Congress, Confederate 9, 10, 11, 162; *see also* legislation, Confederate
Conrad, Daniel B. 22, 30, 79–80, 138, 162, 181, 189; caring for wounded 100–101, 105–6, 125–26; as fleet surgeon 54–55, 83, *84*; as prisoner 105–6; in USS *Underwriter* raid 171, *172*
contract surgeons 69–75
Cook, James V. 117, 191
Cooper, Samuel 17, 161
Cornick, James 15, 27–28, 76, 82, 127, 189; on examining boards 34, 40, 159
courts 166–68
Cowdery, Jonathan 14–15
Crowell, Nathaniel S. 113, 132
cruisers 89–90; *see also specific vessels*
Cushing, William B. 174

Dabney, Flemming 129
CSS *Dalman* 65, 69, 160
Daniel, George C. 176, 193
CSS *Danube* 160
Danville, VA 79, 175–76, 178
Darby, Ralph 71, 160
Davega, Columbus 138
Davidson, John E.A. 117
Davis, Charles H. 3
Davis, George 122
Davis, Jefferson 9, 52, 60, 79, 113, 175, 178
DeBree, John, Jr. (medical officer) 117, 129, 179, 191
DeBree, John, Sr. (paymaster) 121
De Leon, Thomas Cooper 18
Denbigh (steamer) 120
dentistry 154–55
diarrhea 96, 147–48
Dickinson, Luther R. 46, 129, 191
Doucing, Dr. (physician on floating battery) 138
Dowden, George 115, 117
Doyle, Francis 18
CSS *Drewry* 86
Drewry, Samuel D. 33, 47, 85, 160, 191
Drewry's Bluff, VA 85–86, 113, 151, 162, 167–68, 171, 176, 179; batteries 42, 65, 77, *86*, 130, 139; hospital 85–86, 137, 139
drugs *see* medicines

232

Index

Duffel, John E. 129, 191
Dunlop, William 164
Dunnington, John W. 89
Durano, John 104
dysentery 104, 147–48

Edmunds, Nicholas C. *84*, 85, 191
education, medical 35–36, 46
Edwards, E. Harleston 96
Elliott, Stephen 175
Emory, Thomas 47, 90, 105, 106, 163, 191
Evans, Catey 133
Evans, E.J. 133
Evans, John W. 64–65, 132–33
Evans, Rose 133
Evans, William (hospital servant) 133
Evans, William E. (lieutenant) *51*
Everitt, A.C. 137
Ewart, David E. 47, 98, 150, 191
Ewell, Richard S. 176
examinations: of cadet candidates 162; for disability 94, 97, 163–65; of medical-officer candidates 34–38, 39–40; of nonmedical-officer candidates 162–63; of recruits 158–61; of supplies 165–66
expeditions 170–74

Fahs, Charles F. 38, 189
Farragut, David G. 2, 3, 105–6
Farrand, Ebenezer 131
Fennell, Charles N. 18
Ferris, Oscar 96
CSS *Fingal* 72, 77, 146
Fitch, William M. 72
fleet surgeons 53–57, 59, 60, 81, 82–83, 195–96
CSS *Florida* (commerce raider) 90, 93–94, 105, 106, 112, 150, 165, 173–74
CSS *Florida* (gunboat) *see* CSS *Selma*
floating hospitals *70*, 138–39, 141, 144
Foote, George A. 87, 174, 191
Ford, Marcellus 72, 104, 123, 192
Ford, Theodosius Bartow 29, 163, 190
Fort Fisher, NC 74, 86, 87, *88*, 136–37, 139
Fort Hindman, AR 87
Fort Jackson, LA 97
Fort Nelson, VA 127
Fort Pender, NC 137
Fort St. Philip, LA 102
Fort Warren, Boston Harbor 28, 105, 106, 107

CSS *Fredericksburg* 83, 92–93, 97
Freeman, Miles J. *51*
Freeman, Robert J. 93, 98, 103, 105, 152–53, 163, 190

CSS *Gaines 84*; medical records 141, 142–43; sickbay 96–97, 101, 104, 148, 149, 152, 153
Galt, Francis L. 24, *51*, 80, 112, 176, 181, 189; service at batteries 83, 86; service on commerce raiders 90, 105
Galveston, TX 120
Garnett, Alexander Y.P. 26, 31
Garnett, Algernon S. 41, 80, 85, 86, 102, 131, 160, 166–68, 170, 190
Garretson, Frederic 31, 39, 40, 133, 165, 181, 190; *see also* Van Bibber, Frederic
CSS *General Polk* 96, 98–99, 103, 141, 148, 152, 154
CSS *Georgia* (floating battery) 72, 77, 160, 163, 206*ch6n*7
Gibbes, Robert Reeve 31, 60, 77, 94, 104, 112, 159, 175, 180, 190; caring for sick and wounded 86, 103, 146, 149, 150–51, 154, 161; at Charleston Naval Hospital 132–33; examination 36–38, 40; as prisoner 105, 106; and U.S. Navy 29, 32, 36–38; writings 29, 105
Gibbons House, Savannah, GA 134–35, 136
CSS *Giraffe* 90
Goldsborough, Edmund K. 85, 97, 176, 192
Goldsborough, L.M. 106
gonorrhea 152–53
Goodloe, A.W. 71
Goodman, M. Waring 131
Gordon (steamer) 154
Gosport, VA *see* Norfolk, VA
Grafton, Joseph D., Jr. 47, 94, 105, 125, 165, 174, 190
Grant, James O. 160, 176, 192
Graves, Henry L. 161
Graves, William W. 88–89, 131, 159, 160, 192
Green, Bennett W. 30, 79, 90, 129, 180, 190
Green, Daniel S. 47, 53–54, 79, 83, 189
Greenhow, James W. B. 27, 166, 189; as fleet surgeon 28, 54, 83, 137; as prisoner 105, 106; treating yellow fever 136, 149–50

233

Index

Greensboro, NC 138, 176, 179
Griggs, William W. 87, 190

Hacklander, F.R. 124
Halford, Nicholas 96
Halifax, NC 81
Hall, Richard 64–65, 129
Hall, Wilburn B. 72
Halstead, George N. 176, 192
Hamilton, John R. 138
Hampton, Jesse 129
Harley, E.L. 119
Harris, Jeptha V. 131, 192
Harris, Thomas 14, 15
Harrison, James F. 19–20, 27, 30, 40, 129, 155, 166, 178, 189
Harrison, John C. 44, 47, 168, 192
Harrison, William D. 41, 83, 97, 162, 165, 166, 176, 189
USS *Hartford* 101, 107
Hasenburg, F. 71
Havana, Cuba 120
Hays, Archer 73
Hays, Charles W. 117
Helm, Charles J. 120
Henderson, C.R. 73
Henderson, Nathaniel K. 192
Herndon, B.S. 71
Herrick, Stephen S. 81, 181, 192
Herty, James W. 38, 90, 115, 190
Hewlett, C.W. 129
Hicks, James M. 87, 192
Hill, William H. 69, 71, 137
Hollins, George N. 67, 73, 167–68, 170
Horner, G.R.B. 95
hospital stewards 62–68, 82
hospitals, army 78–70, 123, 127, 132, 133, 135, 147, 174; Fort Fisher, NC 87, *88*, 138; Post of Arkansas, AR 87–88, 138; for smallpox 129–30, 151
hospitals, civilian 123–24; Charity, New Orleans, LA 123, 143–44; City (Poor House), Savannah, GA 133–34; Soldier's Home (Ladies), Columbus, GA 104, 123
hospitals, marine 133, 134, 213*n*2
hospitals, naval 123–39; Benton, MS 132; Charleston, SC 64, 98, 132–33, 139, 150, 161; Charlotte, NC 133, 137; Drewry's Bluff, VA 85–86, 137, 139; Fort Fisher, NC 87, *88*, 136–37, 139; Greensboro, NC 138; Mobile, AL 66, 130–32, 152; Norfolk, VA 126–28, 131, 139, 174, 185; Pensacola, FL 18, 106, 124–26, 128, 139, 185; Post of Arkansas, AR 87–88, 138, 139; Richmond, VA 19, 64, 86, 97, 128–30, 151; Roanoke Island, NC 137; Savannah, GA 22, 64, 72, 96, 98, 133–36; ships *70*, 138–39, 141, 144; Smithville, NC 42, 65, 136–37; Wilmington, NC 136–37; *see also* sickbay
Howell, Becket K. *51*
Howell, William F. 122
Huger, Benjamin 127
Hunter, William H. 83, 173
CSS *Huntress* 72, 113
Hynde, M.S. 104

ice 129, 154
Iglehart, Osborn S. 37, 190, 204*n*10; at Battle of Mobile Bay, AL *84*, 101; caring for sick and wounded 96, 104, 144–45, 147, 148, 149, 152, 153; record-keeping 142–43, 147
illness 94–98, 140–57; *see also specific illnesses*
CSS *Indian Chief* 160, 161
Ingraham, Duncan N. 77, 133
instruments, surgical 17–18, *63*, 99, 109, 110, 112, 118–19, 153, 154
Invalid Corps 163–64
CSS *Isondiga* 22, 72
CSS *Ivy* 67

Jackson, Thomas J. "Stonewall" 80
Jeffery, Richard W. 28, 38, 138, 179, 189; at Office of Medicine and Surgery, 19, 21, 22; at Savannah, GA 135, 175
Johnson's Island, OH 173
Johnston, David S. 72
Johnston, G. Floyd 69, 160
Johnston, James D. 69
Johnston, Joseph E. 176
Johnston, Oscar F. 160
Jones, E. Holt 73, 105
Jones, John Pembroke 163
Jones, Thomas M. 125
Jones, William C. 171, 192
Joynes, Levin Smith 130

Kanawha Valley (steamer) 139
USS *Kearsarge* 90, *102*, 103
Kell, John M. *51*, 90
King, Joel G. 122, 129, 192

234

Index

Koch, L. 119
Kuykendall, Robert C. 137, 192

Ladies Hospital, Columbus, GA 104, 123
CSS *Lady Davis* 31, 72, 77, 112, 175
Land, Henry G. 165, 192
Lapwing (bark) 173–74
Lecky, Robert 115, 117, 118, 145
Lee, George Washington Custis 176
Lee, Robert E. 78, 175
Lee, Sidney Smith 83, 161, 168
legislation, Confederate 13, 24, 26, 28, 33, 38–39, 42, 55–60, 122, 160–61, 163–64
Letterman, Jonathan 155
Levin, Dominic 104
Leyburn, John 166, 192
Lincoln, Abraham 9, 109
Lindsay, James E. 28, 37, 38, 85, 90, 130, 190
Lining, Charles E. 25, 81, 85, *180*, 190; caring for sick and wounded 152, 153, 154–55; and CSS *Shenandoah* 90, 156–57, 181
Lining, Thomas 113
Lipscomb, John P. 93, 176, 192
Little Rock, AR 81
CSS *Livingston* 67
Llewellyn, David Herbert 74, 90, 103
CSS *Louisiana* 2, 105
Lowndes, Charles, Jr. 32
Lyles, William D. 124
Lynah, Arthur M. 24, 83, 89, 189, 202n2
Lynch, William F. 54

Macon, GA 34, 39, 159, 179
Maffitt, John N. 150
Major, J.J. 163
malaria 142–47
Mallory, Stephen R. 6, 9–10, *11*, 66, 72, 106, 167–68, 174–75, 182; appointment of medical officers 25–26, 28–29, 38, 41–44, 46; assignment of medical officers 54, 76, 79, 80, 83, 161; flight from Richmond 175, 178; grade and rank of medical officers 57–58, 61; medical purveying 113, 115, 121, 122; organization of Navy Department 13–15, 18, 21, 124
Maloney, Michael 104
CSS *Manassas* 67, 68
Manchester, VA 129
Marine Corps, Confederate 10

Marvin, William 179
Mason, John T. 30, 159, 189
Mason, Randolph F. 30, 47, 126, 189
USS *Massachusetts* 89
CSS *Maurepas* 89
McBride, Raphael 66
McCauley, C.S. 126
McClenahan, William F. 30, 164–65, 189
McGuire, Hunter Holmes 80
McIntosh Bluff, AL 81
McNulty, Frederick J. 74, 156–57
CSS *McRae* 64, 71, 89, 102
McWilkie, Robert H.F. 131
Meade, Hodijah B. 47, 192
Medical College of Virginia 21, 35, 46, 130
medical officers, Confederate 189–94; assisting army 78–80; in battle 98–103; in courts 166–68; deaths 47, duties 76–104, 195–98; examination 34–38, 39–40; on expeditions and raids 170–74; fleet surgeons 53–57, 59, 60, 81, 82–83, 195–96; grades 14, 24, 28, 33, 39–40, 41–44, 200n2; numbers 32, 46–47; origin 28–29, 32, 189–94; postwar activity 180–81; as prisoners 77, 87, 88, 105–7; promotion 38–40; rank 49–52, 56–59, 200n2; salary 52–55, 60; surgeons of station 53–54, 56, 59, 81–82; surrender 176, 179; uniforms 50, *51*, *159*
medical officers, U.S. examination of 34–35, 36–37, 39–40; joining Confederate navy 25–28; numbers 47
medical purveying 108–122; Charleston, SC 111, 113, 114, 115; Mobile, AL 115, 119, 120; New Orleans, LA 112, 119, 120; Savannah, GA 112, 115, 119, 122; Wilmington, NC 111, 114, 115, 120, 187
medicines 108–110; alcohol 121–22; allopathic vs. sectarian 35, 141; antimonial wine 149; "black wash" 154; boneset 118, 145–46; calcined magnesia 149; castor oil 148; chloroform 99, *100*, 101; colchicum seed 148–49; corn meal 147; Dover's powder 148, 149; ether 99, 101; fodder tea 147; Fowler's solution 146; gum arabic 149; hemp 146; lead acetate 147; lobelia 118, 149; mercury 148, 152; nitric acid 152; opiates 99, 147–48, 149, 152, 154;

Index

potassium arsenite 146; potassium iodide 148; quinine 108, 109, 119–20, 144–46, seneka 149; silver nitrate 152; squill 117, 149; zinc 152
Melvin, Henry B. 85, 176, 190
CSS *Merrimack* (*Virginia*) 65, 79, 87, 102
USS *Michigan* 173
Minor, Lewis W. *30*, 34, 64, 129, 189; at Norfolk, VA 126, 127; as surgeon of station 53–54, 67, 81, 82, 131, 138–39
Minor, R.D. 127
CSS *Mississippi* 2
Mitchell, John K. 50, 51, 83, 97, 143, 165–66
CSS *Mobile* 67, 68, 71
Mobile, AL 66, 78, 96, 154, 165, 181; hospital 66, 130–32, 152; medical purveying 115, 119, 120; naval station 53, 69, 81, 82, 141; receiving ship 160; rendezvous 159; squadron 43, 53, 54, 59, 83, *84*, 86, 97, 141, 142, 144, 145, 168
Mobile Bay, AL 65, 88, 142, 154
USS *Monitor* 174
Montgomery, AL 9, 17, 112
Monticello, FL 115
Moore, Samuel Preston 19, 21, 45, 46, 78, 117–18, 145, 178–79
Morfit, Charles M. 29, 30, 32, 40, 60, 81, 105, 114, 115, 118, 190
CSS *Morgan* 54, 66, *84*
Morgan, George 65
Moyler, James Edward 166, 176, 192
Murdaugh, William H. *180*

CSS *Nashville* 74
Nassau, Bahamas 90, 111, 180
naval stations 53, 80–81; Charleston, SC 77, 81, 114, 176; Halifax, NC 81; Mobile, AL 53, 69, 81, 82, 141; New Orleans, LA 67, 81, 139; Richmond, VA 78, 79, 80, 141; St. Marks, FL 115, 117; Savannah, GA 81, 175; Wilmington, NC 176
navies, state 25, 29–31, 127
navy, Confederate 18, *20*; organization 13, 18, 200n1; personnel 10, 49, 140–41; Provisional Navy of the Confederate States 42–44, 52, 60; receiving ships *70*, 158, 160, 161, 163; *see also* naval stations; navy yards; Office of Medicine and Surgery (Confederate); Office of Orders and Detail; squadrons
navy, U.S. 13–15, 34–35, 62–64; Naval laboratory 110, 114; as source of Confederate naval medical officers 24–29, 31–32, 34
navy yards 62–63, 65, 68, 80–82; Charlotte, NC 137, 164, 182; Little Rock, AR 81; McIntosh Bluff, AL 81; Oven Bluff, AL 81; Pee Dee, SC 81; Pensacola, FL 9, 18, 65, 81; Richmond, VA 129; Saffold, GA 72, 81; Wilmington, NC 136–37; Yazoo City, MS 132
CSS *Neuse* 122
CSS *New Orleans* 67–68
New Orleans, LA 33, 71, 73; Charity Hospital 123, 143–44; medical purveying 112, 119, 120; naval station 67, 81, 139; rendezvous 159; CSS *St. Philip* 138, 141, 144, 160; squadron 67
USS *Niagara* 79
Norfolk, VA 126, 175; hospital 126–28, 131, 139, 174, 185; receiving ship 160, rendezvous 159
CSS *North Carolina* 137
nurses 63, 124–25, 129, 133, 136, 214n17

CSS *Oconee* 105
Office of Medicine and Surgery (Confederate) 13–14, 15–22, 81, 94, 183–84, 186–87; publications 112, 201n16; reports 18; staff 18–10, 77, 78
Office of Orders and Detail 13, 50, 54, 82, 83
Office of Provisions and Clothing 13, 121, 122
Ould, Robert 129
Oven Bluff, AL 81

Page, William M. 28, 120, 179, 189
Paisley, Hugh S. 45, 81, 192
CSS *Palmetto State* 93
Paris, France 112
Parker, Cincinnatus M. 46, 83, 161, 190
Parker, Francis F. 67
Parker, William H. 99
CSS *Patrick Henry* 77, 86, 93, 139, 146, 162–64, 164–65
Patton (steamer) 139
Patton, William F. 30, 81, 114, 127, 132, 179, 189
Peck, Frederick 176, 192
Pee Dee, SC 81
Pegram, Robert B. 168
Pelaez, Charles 67
Pelot, James M. 30

236

Index

Pelzer, F.J. 132
USS *Pennsylvania* 126
Pensacola, FL 78, 124; hospital 18, 106, 124–26, 128, 139, 185; navy yard 9, 18, 65, 81; and W.A.W. Spotswood 16–17, 18, 19, 179, 181
personnel, Confederate marines 10
personnel, Confederate navy 10, 49, 140–41
Peyton, Griffin 129
Phillips, Dinwiddie B. 30, 78–79, 102, 146–47, 162, 174–75, 181, 190
Pierson, W.H. 102–3, 135, 173
Plymouth, NC 174
Polk, Leonidas 175
CSS *Pontchartrain* 81, 87
Poor House Hospital, Savannah, GA 72, 133–34
Porcher, Francis Peyre 118, 127
Port Walthall Junction, VA 86
Portsmouth, VA *see* Norfolk, VA
Post, Christopher Columbus 67
Post of Arkansas, AR 87–88, 138, 139
Potts, Richard 113
Powell, Robert C. 131, 192
prisoners, Confederate 77, 87, 88, 105–7
prisoners, Union 185
Provisional Navy of the Confederate States 42–44, 52, 60
Purcell, Ladd and Company 113, 118, 129, 146, 149

Quincy, FL 117
quinine 108, 109, 119–20, 144–46
Quitman, GA 115

raids 170–74
CSS *Raleigh* 166
Raleigh, NC 159
rank 49–52, 56–59, 200*n*2
CSS *Rappahannock* 71, 90, 112
Read, Charles W. 102
Read, Nathaniel M. 81, 88, 192
receiving ships *70*, 158, 160, 161, 163
USS *Red Rover* 3
USS *Reliance* 173
rendezvous, naval 76, 77, 80, 82, 119, 158–60; Charleston, SC 119, 159; Mobile, AL 159; Norfolk, VA 159; Richmond, VA 82, 159; Savannah, GA 77, 159
CSS *Resolute* 72, 105
rheumatism 148–49

CSS *Richmond* 166
USS *Richmond* 107
Richmond, VA 19, 93; education in 21, 46; evacuation 175–76; examination of medical officers or candidates 34, 40; fire 178, *183*; government buildings 18, *20*, 178, *183*; hospitals 19, 64, 86, 97, 128–30, 151; medical purveying 112, 113–19, 146–47, 186–87; naval rendezvous 82, 159; naval station 78, 79, 80, 141; Office of Medicine and Surgery 81
Ritter, William 128
Roanoke Island, NC 137
CSS *Robert E. Lee* 90
Robertson, F.H. 118
Ross and Ketchum 131
Rutherford, John B. 135, 193

Sabarino, Francisco 104
Saffold, GA 72, 81
St. Charles, AR 89
St. Marks, FL 115, 117
St. Nicholas (steamer) 168, 170
CSS *St. Philip* *70*, 71, 123, 138–39, 141, 144, 160
Sale, William D. 46, 176, 193
CSS *Sampson* 72, 77, 160
Samuel Orr (steamer) 139
Sandford, John W., Jr. 39, 81, 137, 190
Sands, Andrew H. 168
USS *Satellite* 173
CSS *Savannah* 72, 77, 82–83, 97, 150–51
Savannah, GA *128*, 154; hospital 22, 64, 72, 96, 98, 133–36; hospital ship 139; medical purveying 112, 115, 119, 122; naval station 81, 175; receiving ship 97, 160; rendezvous 77, 159; squadron 83, 96, 98, 141, 143, 150, 163
Scott, William 65
scurvy 153
CSS *Seabird* 72, 105
seasickness 154
CSS *Selma* 73, *84*, 105, 119, 168, 181
Semmes, Raphael *51*, 74, 90, 153, 175–76
Semmes's Naval Brigade 175–76
sexually transmitted diseases 152–53
CSS *Shenandoah* 74, 90, 152, 153, 154, 156, 181
Sheppardson, William 85, 160, 173, 193
Shepperd, Francis E. 71
Shepperd, John J. 131
Sheridan, Philip 107
Ship Island, MS 89

Index

sickbay **63**, 94–98
Sinclair, Arthur, Jr. 90
Sinclair, William B. 19, 21, 30, 40, 73, 126, 155, 159, 166, 190
smallpox 72, 129–30, 150–51, 160
Smith, Howard 113
Smith, Ira E. 193
Smith, Jacob 67
Smithfield, NC 42, 65, 136–37
Soldier's Home Hospital, Columbus, GA 104, 123
Spikes, W.B. 65
spirit ration 121–22, 155–56
Spotswood, Dillon Jordan 17
Spotswood, George Willis 16–17
Spotswood, Mary Eastin 17, 181
Spotswood, Mary G. 17
Spotswood, Thomas Eastin 17
Spotswood, William A.W. 15, 16–23, 124, 125, 178–79, 181, 182–84, 190; appointment of medical officers 24, 28, 32, 41–44; assignment of medical officers 76, 81, 82, 92, 187–88; establishment of hospitals 129, 137, 138; medical purveying 113–120, 145, 186–87; own grade and rank 52, 54–55; recommendations on caring for sick and wounded 141–43, 155, 166
CSS *Spray* 117
squadrons 81, 82–83, 204*n*23; Charleston, SC 83, 98, 115, 176; James River, VA 53, 59, 83, 92, 97, 130, 139, 141, 143, 155, 165–66, 175–76; Mississippi River 67, 71, 123, 141; Mobile, AL 43, 53–54, 59, 83, **84**, 86, 97, 141, 142, 144–45, 168; North Carolina 54, 59, 83, 87, 99, 137, 139, 176; Savannah, GA 83, 96, 98, 141, 143, 150, 163
Stanbery, Henry 179
Stanton, Edwin 173
Star of the West see CSS *St. Philip*
state navies 25, 29–31, 127
stations *see* naval stations
Stedman, Charles Ellery **37**, **100**, **156**
Steele, Thomas B. 32
Steinriede, John Joseph 47, 67, 132, 193
Stephens, F.W. 31
stewards, surgeons' and hospital 62–68, 82; physicians as 66–68
Stoakley, William S. 135, 161, 173, 190
Stone, Henry 47, 193
CSS *Stonewall* 90, 180
CSS *Stono* 115

Stribling, John M. **51**
CSS *Sumter* **51**, 71, 90, 112, 153
supplies 108–122
surgeons *see* medical officers, Confederate; medical officers, U.S.
surgeons of station 53–54, 56, 59, 81–82
surgeons' stewards 62–68, 82
surveys: for disability 97, 163–65; of equipment or supplies 165–66
Sussdorff, Gustave E. 176, 193
syphilis 152

CSS *Tallahassee* 117
Tatnall, Josiah 150, 175
CSS *Tennessee* **84**, 100, 105, 107
Texas Marine Department 31
Thom, R.T. 89
Thomas, C. Wesley 102, 171, 176, 190
Thomas, James Grey 45, 193
Thomas, Richard 170
Tipton, Joseph S. 47, 105, 190
tooth decay 154–55
CSS *Torpedo* 71
Toucey, Isaac 26
tourniquets 99, **119**, 171, 197
Trent, Peterfield 146
Trimble, Isaac R. 80
Tucker, John H. (medical officer) 179, 193
Tucker, John R. (captain) 176
Tucker's Brigade 176
Turner, John 66
Turner, William Mason 46, 85, 119, 179, 193
CSS *Tuscaloosa* 181

USS *Underwriter* 171, **172**
CSS *United States* 160
Upshur, Abel P. 14

Van Benthuysen, Alfred C. 167–68
Van Bibber, Frederic 30, 112, 190; *see also* Garretson, Frederic
Venable, Howell A. 176, 193
CSS *Virginia* 65, 79, 87, 102
CSS *Virginia II* 42, 83, 165

Waddell, James I. 74
Wakefield, F.B. 72
Wallace, Robert 64–65
Walters, John 96
Ward, John 24, 47, 190
Ware, Thomas R. 120

Index

Warley, A. F. 89
Warner, Watkins L. 193
Warren, Edward 31
Warrington, FL *see* Pensacola, FL
Washington, Henry W.M. 30, 72, 81, 83, 92, 136, 166, 190
USS *Water Witch* 102–3, 135, 171, 174
Waterman, George S. *84*, 85, 88
Weston, George B. 193
Wharton, Mrs. (slave owner) 129
Wheeden, Thomas J. 90, 179, 193
Whelan, William 14–15, 124, 125, 127
Whittle, William C. 139
Williams, John Q.A. 65
Williams, William T. 47, 193
Williamson, Charles H. 27, 30, 82–83, 126, 137, 190

Wilmington, NC 87, *116*; hospital 136–37; medical purveying 111, 114, 115, 120, 187; naval station 176, navy yard 136–37; receiving ship 160, squadron 54, 59, 83, 87, 99, 137, 139, 176
Wingfield, A.C. 123
Wise, Henry A. 78
women 19, 119, 123
Wood, John Taylor 173
wounded, treatment of 98–104
Wysham, M.E. 131
Wysham, William E. 30, 120, 126, 131, 190

Yazoo City, MS 132
yellow fever 98, 149–50

www.ingramcontent.com/pod-product-compliance
Lightning Source LLC
Chambersburg PA
CBHW032039300426
44117CB00009B/1114